MISSY VINEYARD is one of the foremost master teachers of the Alexander Technique in the United States today. Vineyard is director of the Alexander Technique School New England (ATSNE), a three-year teacher-training program that she founded in 1987, and the author of numerous articles. In 1987 she cofounded AmSAT, the national professional society for Alexander teachers in the United States, and served as its first chairman. For the last twenty years she has devoted much of her schedule to teacher and postgraduate training, and to developing a unique, systematic curriculum for imparting the subtle hands-on skill that is the hallmark of the Alexander teacher. She maintains a busy private teaching practice, specializing in working with performing artists and children to enhance their artistic and athletic performance. Vineyard has two sons and two stepdaughters, and lives with her husband and two standard poodles in Amherst, Massachusetts.

To learn more or contact Missy Vineyard, visit her Web site at www.missyvineyard.com.

MISSY VINEYARD

Learning the Alexander Technique to Explore Your Mind-Body Connection and Achieve Self-Mastery

HOW YOU STAND, HOW YOU MOVE, HOW YOU LIVE

with illustrations by Matthew Mitchell

MARLOWE & COMPANY
NEW YORK

HOW YOU STAND, HOW YOU MOVE, HOW YOU LIVE:
Learning the Alexander Technique to Explore Your Mind-Body Connection and Achieve Self-Mastery
Copyright © 2007 by Missy Vineyard
Illustrations copyright © 2007 by Matthew Mitchell

Published by
Marlowe and Company
An Imprint of Avalon Publishing Group, Incorporated
245 West 17th Street • 11th Floor
New York, NY 10011–5300

AVALON
publishing group incorporated

Some of the material in this book has been published in somewhat different form in *AmSAT News*.

The information in this book is intended to help readers make informed decisions about their health and the health of their loved ones. It is not intended to be a substitute for treatment by or the advice and care of a professional health care provider. While the authors and publisher have endeavored to ensure that the information presented is accurate and up to date, they shall not be held responsible for loss or damage of any nature suffered as a result of reliance on any of this book's contents or any errors or omissions herein.

ISBN-13: 978-1-60094-006-4

Designed by Pauline Neuwirth, Neuwirth & Associates, Inc.

Printed in the United States of America

*In memory of my teachers
Judith Leibowitz and
Walter Carrington,*

*for my sons
Jared and Jules,*

and

*for Tommy,
the light of my life*

CONTENTS

Table of Illustrations   xiii

I. Introduction   1

II. Introduction to the Alexander Technique   7

III. Introduction to the Self-Experiments   12

PART 1: HOW DO YOU MOVE? Tales from the Beginning   15

1. Surprising Observations   17

    John, Part One   17

2. A Malfunctioning Locomotor System   23

    Erin, Part One   23

3. How Did We Get This Way? From Fish to
    Horse to Biped   27

4. Standing on Two Legs: The Biped's Challenge   35

    SELF-EXPERIMENTS   41

    A. Rest Your Back   41

      Semisupine   42

      Prone   45

    B. Motion and Mind   48

      How You Move   48

      Can You Change?   51

      Noticing Your Habit   52

      Your Mind-Body Connection   53

PART 2: HOW DO YOU FEEL? The Mind-Body Link   55

5. A Sense of Feeling   57

6. Feelings Gone Wrong   64

    Gary   64

    Betty, Part One   67

7. The Feeling of Fear   71

    How We Perceive Danger   73

8. Fear's Body–Mind   77
    In the Grip of Fear   77
    A Threatening Injury   80
    The Shrinking World of Pain   83
9. Anxiety and Performance   91
    Bruce, Part One   91
10. Attention, Awareness, and Conscious Inhibition   99
    Bruce, Part Two   99

PART 3: HOW DO YOU THINK? The Mind Changes Everything   105

11. A Fine Day in London with Nothing to Feel   107
12. Discovering the Thinking Mind   111
    The Attic   115
    Surprises and Beliefs   121
13. Believing Is Not Seeing   128
14. The Difference that Inhibition Makes   137
    Erin, Part Two   137
15. You Have a Helper   145

    SELF-EXPERIMENTS   151
    C. How to Inhibit   151
        Quiet Your Inner Conversation   152
        Turn on Your Prefrontal Cortex   155
        Think with Meaning   160
        The Positive "No"   164
        Conscious Inhibition   166
    D. Acts of Inhibition   168
        Stop Moving   168
        Think of Not Doing   169
        Let Your Helper Do It   170
        Let Go of Belief   172

PART 4: SPACE AND DIRECTION: Our Hidden Sense   175

16. Fewer Words, More Space   177
    Cleo   179
    Meghan   187

17. More Problems with Feelings   189
    Nathan   190
    Nancy   193
18. Balance and Coordination   197
19. A New Way of Moving   210
    Brian   210
    Betty, Part Two   212

SELF-EXPERIMENTS   217
    E. How to Direct   217
        Think of a Cube   218
        Up-Down, Wide, Forward-Back   218
        Putting Directions Together   220
        Turning Your Head   222
        Forward and Up   223
        Thinking Names of Body Parts   224
        Alexander's Directions   225
    F. Moving with Inhibition and Direction   228
        Bending Your Leg   228
        Moving Forward and Back   229
        Standing and Sitting   232

PART 5: TOUCH: Our Forgotten Sense   233

20. Touching the Heart   235
    Sam   235
    What Is It about Touch?   237
21. The Teacher's Hands   245

PART 6: CONSCIOUSNESS: Our Newest Sense   261

22. Pain Free and Moving Again   263
    John, Part Two   263
23. An Incredible Lightness of Being   270
    Erin, Part Three   270
24. Speaking from My Self   277
    Greg   277
25. Self-Mastery: Connection   285

SELF-EXPERIMENTS   289

   G. How to Strengthen Your Back   289

      Neck Extensors   290

      Neck and Back Extensors   293

   H. Self-Mastery Every Day   295

      Exercise   296

      Sports   298

      Practice and Performance   299

      Anxiety   300

      Pain   301

      How You Live   302

Appendix: How to Find a Teacher   305

Glossary   306

Notes   311

Bibliography   313

Acknowledgments   316

Index   318

FIGURES

II-1.	Woman with neck forward, head back	8
II-2.	Woman with neck back, head forward and down	9
II-3.	Woman with neck back, head forward and up	10
1-1.	John sitting	18
1-2.	John raising arm	22
2-1.	Erin sitting	25
2-2.	Erin starting to stand up	25
3-1.	Evolution of vertebrate locomotor systems	29
3-2.	Progression of human infant motor development	30
3-3.	Schema for placement of center of gravity of head, torso, legs	32
3-4.	Standing skeleton with good use	33
4-1.	Standing skeleton with bad use	37
4-2.	John walking	38
4-3.	Erin walking	39
A-1-1.	Semisupine: head on books	42
A-1-2.	Semisupine: no books under head, neck arched	43
A-1-3.	Semisupine: no books under head, neck flattened	43
A-1-4.	Semisupine: too many books under head	44
A-1-5.	Semisupine: pillows under legs	44
A-2-1.	Prone	45
A-2-2.	Prone: books under chest	46
A-2-3.	Prone: no books under chest	46
B-1-1.	Standing: hand on back of head and neck.	49
B-1-2.	Starting to sit: hand on back of head and neck	49
B-1-3.	Starting to stand: hand on back of head and neck	49
6-1.	Betty starting to step while collapsing on standing leg	68
8-1.	Face of fear: Attack	87
8-2.	Face of fear: Withdrawer	87
8-3.	Face of fear: Freeze	87
8-4.	Face of fear: Submit	87
9-1.	Bruce playing piano with head and neck tension	92
10-1.	Bruce playing piano without head and neck tension	101

12-1.	Semisupine: bending leg with unnecessary muscle tension	117
12-2.	Semisupine: bending leg while inhibiting, preventing unnecessary tension	120
14-1.	Erin standing habitually	138
14-2.	Erin sitting down with guidance from teacher	141
14-3.	Erin sitting with guidance from teacher	141
14-4.	Erin moving backward in chair with habitual tension	143
16-1.	Facial expression without thinking spatially	186
16-2.	Facial expression while thinking spatially	186
17-1.	Nancy balancing on one leg with habitual tension	194
18-1.	Vertical up (A), and headward up (B)	201
18-2.	Baby sitting	206
18-3.	Dog sitting relaxed	207
18-4.	Dog sitting with headward up coordination	207
19-1.	Betty starting to step while inhibiting and directing	215
23-1.	Erin sitting with improved balance and coordination	274
23-2.	Erin standing with improved balance and coordination	276
G-1-1.	Prone: lifting neck with neck extensors	290
G-1-2.	Prone: lifting head with head extensors	291
G-2-1.	Prone: lifting neck and upper body with neck and back extensors	294

Introduction

Make the most of yourself,
for that is all there is of you.
—R. W. EMERSON

THERE IS A poster of Michael Jordan on the wall in my teaching room that I like to show my students. Jordan is four feet off the ground, suspended in the air halfway between the foul line from which he has departed and the basket toward which he is aiming and soon to dunk the ball. He is as close to a human bird as I have seen—a massive, four-limbed bird in improbable flight. There are many striking aspects to this picture: Jordan's height in the air; the distance he has traveled and has yet to travel, airborne, en route to the basket; his strong, upright torso. Most astonishing is the expression on his face. It is apparent that his mind is not focused on his body. He is not feeling what his legs are doing, checking out where his arms are going, or wondering where he will land. His mind is focused on the basket as every part of his body fulfills his purpose in easy and fluid coordination, following the direction of his mind's intent.

"Wow! How does he do that?" my students ask in a tone of wonder. The next question is spoken slowly, with a distant note of self-reproach: "Why can't I do that?"

It is my job to answer their questions, but I am not a basketball coach, exercise trainer, or sports psychologist. Nor are my students necessarily athletes. They are anyone and everyone. They come from all ages, backgrounds, and occupations, and they come for many reasons. I teach the Alexander Technique—a method that explores *how* you do what you do.

The Alexander Technique teaches you to improve your movement skill in activities such as standing, sitting, walking, running, lifting, playing an instrument, hitting a ball, jumping. It teaches you to reduce unnecessary tension and to move with balance and coordination. More important, by learning to improve how you use your body, you also learn to improve how you use your mind. The Alexander Technique teaches you to better understand yourself, physically and mentally. This deeper self-knowledge becomes a tool that lets you play a greater part in recovering from injury, maintaining health, improving posture, learning new skills, aging gracefully, and achieving a deeper sense of well-being. Whatever your age, whatever your background and interests, the Alexander Technique lets you explore your mind-body connection to help you achieve self-mastery.

For example, how do you stand? Do your feet turn out or point straight ahead? Are your shoulders pulled back, or forward, or lifted? How does your head sit on top of your neck? Is it tilted backward or forward? Is it rotated? Do you stand the way your best friend does? Do you stand efficiently, with almost no effort in your muscles and an easy lightness throughout your body? Or do you stand with your knees locked, pelvis pushed forward, spine compressed, and jaw clenched? How did you learn to stand? Do you know whether this is important? Perhaps you find such questions bewildering. You just stand. You do not think about it. What more is there to say? In fact, there is a great deal to say, observe, and learn.

This book explores how you stand and, by extension, how you do anything you do. This means we will look at how you use your mind, how you use your body, and how they interact to create your behavior. We will approach this topic by learning about a method developed at the turn of the last century by F. M. Alexander, known today around the world as the Alexander Technique. Alexander was an actor with a vocal problem. To recover his voice, he did a simple thing. He studied himself in a mirror and made important discoveries about how our thoughts and movements are bound together to create our unconscious and **habitual way of moving** that can lead to injury, undermine our health, and limit what we are able to learn and accomplish. Then he discovered how we can bring our thoughts and movements to a conscious level and tease them apart to enhance both how we think and how we move.

Today, more than fifty years since his death, people all over the world and from all walks of life are learning Alexander's method of self-study to improve how they function. Well-known past and current students of the Technique include John Dewey, George Bernard Shaw, Aldous Huxley, Kevin Kline, William Hurt, Mary Steenburgen, Renée Fleming, and Robertson Davies. Alexander teachers are employed at many of the leading performing arts schools around the world, including Juilliard, NYU, UCLA, and London's Royal Academy of Dramatic Arts.

Since you cannot experience this hands-on method by reading about it, I have done the next closest thing. I have compiled a collection of true stories drawn from more than thirty years of teaching experience to show you this learning process in action. You will meet John, who suffers from a frozen shoulder, and Erin, who has chronic back pain that prevents her from playing tennis. You will meet Bruce, a pianist with performance anxiety, and Ed, who suffers from inexplicable arm pain. You will meet Nancy, a dancer who has trouble balancing on one leg; Nathan, a teenager who wants to improve his pitching; Joan, who is virtually paralyzed by fear; and Greg, an actor with a flat and stilted voice.* These and other stories show students learning the Alexander Technique as they acquire the skills to change lifelong patterns of mental and physical behavior that have been undermining how they function.

In addition to the stories, the book draws from my personal study of the Technique and from recent research in neuroscience to shed light on what Alexander discovered but could not fully explain. The book breaks new ground as it probes deeply into the two essential but little-known cognitive skills that are central to the method: **inhibition**, a type of thinking that prevents unwanted tension, unnecessary emotional reaction, and maladaptive behavior; and

---

* All students' names and physical characteristics have been changed to protect their privacy (with the exception of my sons). The students represented in the illustrations are personal friends who kindly agreed to model for the artist.

direction, a type of spatial thinking that enhances our balance and coordination as we move. The book discusses the physiological basis of these skills and how they improve physical performance and brain functioning.

The book also includes a series of Self-Experiments that allow you to explore your mind–body connection to discover how your mind and body connect and interact, and that teach you the skills for self-mastery. You will learn to rest your back and strengthen your back muscles; observe your movement habits in action; inhibit and direct; and apply your new cognitive skills in simple and everyday activities.

Since this is an Introduction, I will not yet venture into the subject of how you stand, or precisely how you do the things you do, but begin instead with a question: Have you ever noticed that, even though you have been making decisions about moving your body throughout your day, virtually every day of your life, you do not know very much about how you do this? How does a mere thought trigger nerves to send their electrochemical signals, so that a simple decision (I want to stand) becomes a physical act (I am standing)?

Although this question might be approached through complicated explanations of neurological functioning and muscle anatomy, I am going to offer you a simple metaphor: How you move—*the way that you do what you do*—is information that is locked away in a black box within you, hidden beneath your conscious awareness. It is so hidden from view that you do not even realize you lack this understanding—not on a scientific level—but on a level of simple self-observation and awareness. Nor are you likely to notice this essential mystery within yourself until, one day, you experience a problem such as an injury, chronic pain, or some other physical or psychological limitation that prevents you from being able to do what you want to do.

Perhaps one day you bent down to pick up a sock and felt a sudden, stabbing pain in your lower back and crumpled to the floor. *Why did this happen?* Perhaps when you were young you sat easily at your desk and studied all night, but now, decades later, you often find yourself in pain as you sit at your desk. *Why is this happening now?* Perhaps you are learning to play a musical instrument. Your teacher explains what your fingers and arms must do but you cannot make them obey. It seems impossible to do what you are told to do, despite your sincere efforts. *Why aren't you able to learn to do this?* Perhaps you slipped one day on the ice, falling and breaking your leg. Months later your leg has healed, but whenever you walk any distance you experience pain. *Why doesn't it get better?*

Perhaps you suffer from any of a myriad of musculoskeletal injuries: tendinitis, arthritis, carpal tunnel syndrome, tennis elbow, ruptured disk, or repetitive strain injury, which are not helped very much by pain medication, exercises, or even surgery. *Is there anything else that can be done?* Perhaps you are a musician, dancer, actor, or athlete. You understand that you have learned to move your body in a way that is inefficient and even harmful, but you cannot stop moving in your usual way. *Why is it so difficult to change?*

Once we experience a physical injury, or have difficulty learning a skill, or discover the frustration of not being able to do what we try to do, we start to wonder why this is happening. But finding the answer is not easy. We may begin by seeking help from doctors, psychologists, or other health professionals, but this often means being treated for symptoms rather than addressing their source, or analyzing our behavior rather than learning the skills for change. We may exercise to strengthen specific muscles, but this does not teach us to coordinate our entire body as we move. We may try harder and practice longer, but this does not help us to understand our unconscious, harmful patterns of tension, or how to correct our skewed self-conceptions.

Worse, when our efforts do not succeed, we tell ourselves that we are the way we are because of our fate or genes, resigning ourselves to our problem because we are convinced there is nothing more we can do. Or we assume that our partial self-understanding and limited self-awareness is the best we are capable of, and so believe we cannot search any more deeply into ourselves to find the cause of our problem. Or we are afraid to probe too deeply, fearful of what we will discover.

However, there is an option besides fatalism, passive acceptance, or fearful withdrawal. There is the possibility of finding our hidden box, learning to open it, and peering inside to discover its secrets. Here we find the realm where our thoughts, feelings, actions, and beliefs intermingle. This is the area of dynamic interaction and connection between the many aspects of our selves. It is also the realm of *misconnection,* where the mind misperceives the body's feelings, where the body fails to respond skillfully according to the mind's intent, where misconceptions lead us astray, and where imagined fears stop us in our tracks.

If we can learn to perceive these misconnections, however, we discover that we have been unwittingly creating and/or compounding the problems from which we suffer. Then we are ready to begin learning the skills for restoration and reconnection. With awareness, our conscious mind can become a tool for change. We can consciously learn to shift our perceptions and better understand our feelings. We can consciously learn to perceive our body more accurately and objectively. We can learn to stand and to move with greater efficiency, balance, and coordination. Our body can become better able to do as we intend.

Where is such knowledge and skill to be found? This is the territory into which the Alexander Technique ventures, a method not of self-absorption but of self-understanding; not of treatment and exercise but of skilled, effective bodily control; not of intellectual self-analysis but of experiential learning that teaches us how to identify and release our harmful reactions to pain, fear, and anxiety. The Alexander Technique teaches us to look more deeply into ourselves, and to better operate the self from within. *How You Stand, How You Move, How You Live* shows you how.

II

Introduction to the Alexander Technique

How use doth breed a habit in a man!
—WILLIAM SHAKESPEARE

FREDERICK MATTHIAS ALEXANDER was born in 1869 on the island of Tasmania off the southeast coast of Australia. As an infant he was sickly but grew into a bright, precocious youngster with a tendency to ask too many questions in school. This disrupted the other children, so the local schoolmaster tutored him privately. Alexander's close relationship with his teacher, who loved the theater, was an important influence. As a teen he dreamed of becoming an actor but as the oldest in a large family, he was expected to help with the family finances. At seventeen, Alexander left home and took a job as a bookkeeper at a tin-mining company. But after a few years, his longing for the theater prevailed. Alexander began taking classes in elocution, acting, and violin. Soon he was giving recitals to highly favorable reviews. And then, suddenly, his prospects dimmed when he developed a strange hoarseness in his voice.

Seeking medical help, Alexander's doctor advised him to drink tea with honey and not to speak for several weeks to give his voice a rest. After he followed these instructions his voice improved, but when he returned to performing his hoarseness returned as well.

"Keep drinking tea and honey and resting your voice," his doctor instructed.

"Why should I?" Alexander countered. "My voice gets better when I don't speak but gets hoarse again when I do. Doesn't this suggest that I'm doing something harmful to my voice when I speak?"

His doctor agreed this was a reasonable theory.

"Then why should I keep doing as you suggest? Resting my voice only helps if I don't speak!" The doctor admitted this was a fair point but had nothing more to offer. Unwilling to abandon the new career on which he had staked so much, Alexander resolved to solve his problem himself.

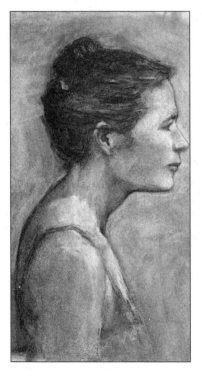

INTRODUCTION II-1.
Woman with poor head-neck coordination: neck jutting forward (excessive neck curvature), head pulled back and down on the neck, and shoulders rounded forward.

Using two mirrors, he watched his profile as he spoke and noticed something surprising. Each time he began to speak, he saw his head move back and downward on his neck as his neck thrust forward, and he gulped awkwardly for air (Illustration II-1). Alexander was not certain if this odd mannerism was related to his vocal problem, but he decided to stop doing it. When he tried, however, he was startled to discover that he could not prevent it. Every time he spoke, this unconscious way of moving reasserted itself. It seemed he had an unconscious way of using his muscles over which he had no control. He could consciously decide to speak or not, but he could not prevent himself from tensing his neck muscles, pulling his head back, and gulping for air as he spoke.

With further observation, Alexander discovered that this way of moving his head and neck acted like a current running through him, accompanying everything he did. He also realized he had not been aware of this tension as it happened because he did not feel it. He concluded that his way of moving was damaging his vocal mechanism. He needed to learn to prevent this, but how?

Reviewing his progress, Alexander realized that he had several unconscious beliefs about his body. He believed that he would know if he was doing something harmful to himself. He believed that as long as he was not sick, his body would function normally. And he believed that, with sufficient practice, he could make his body do what he wanted. But his observations in the mirror disproved them all. He had not felt what he was doing with his neck muscles, and so had not been aware of his tension as he spoke. He had actually been damaging his body by this unconscious tension, causing his hoarseness. And he could not make his body do what he wanted.

Continuing to observe himself in the mirror, Alexander saw that whenever he had a mere thought to speak, this previously unconscious **misuse** of his body reasserted itself. This meant that his *thought of speaking* played a central role in *how he spoke*, which brought to light another wrong belief—that his mind and body were separate. He had assumed that a physical problem arose from his body, and a mental problem arose from his mind. As such, he had believed his hoarseness was a physical problem. But this idea of separation was clearly wrong. He saw in the mirror, unmistakably, that his thought of speaking produced a response of excess tension in his body.

Alexander realized he was trapped in a chicken-and-egg sort of problem. In order to prevent his misuse and restore his voice, he would have to change the whole of himself, mind and body: how he thought and how he moved. But where should he begin?

First, Alexander tried to do the opposite movement with his head and neck. Instead of thrusting his neck forward and pulling his head back, he pushed his neck back and pulled his head forward (Illustration II-2). While this produced a change in his appearance, his voice did not improve. Next he noticed that any change in the way he usually moved his head and neck felt *wrong* to him, while his old way of speaking (which he now understood to be wrong) felt *right*. Not only was he unaware of his tension habit, he could not accurately perceive what his body was doing. His way of speaking was tied to his mind's misinterpretation of physical sensations, warping his judgment. This meant that physical sensation was an all-important bridge, linking his body's movements with his mind's perception. His incorrect self-perception and physical misuse were tied together. He was locked in a vicious cycle of misuse, faulty perception and judgment, and further misuse.

Alexander decided that instead of doing the opposite movement with his head and neck, he would try thinking the opposite thought.

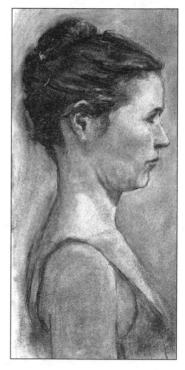

INTRODUCTION II-2.
Woman with poor head-neck coordination: neck pushed back (too little neck curvature), jaw pulled back, head forward and down, and shoulders pulled back.

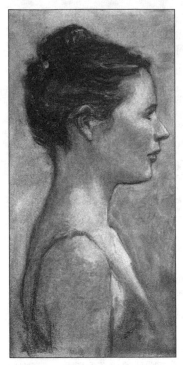

INTRODUCTION II-3.
Woman with skilled head-neck coordination: neck lengthening upward (normal neck curvature), head poised forward and up on top of the neck, jaw suspended freely from the head, and shoulders widening apart.

Since telling himself to speak triggered his faulty way of moving, he tried telling himself *not* to speak. Watching in the mirror as he repeated this self-instruction, Alexander was astonished to see that his muscle tension melted away. His neck lengthened upward. His head shifted *forward and up* on the top of his spine. His spine lengthened and his ribs moved more readily, helping him to breathe (Illustration II-3). Although these changes felt wrong to him, he could see in the mirror that his body appeared more relaxed and more upright, and his head did not pull back and down on his neck.

In neuroscience, *excitation* is the term that refers to the activation of a neuron, which can stimulate a muscle to contract. *Inhibition* is the term that describes the opposite—a signal that causes another neuron not to be activated, thus preventing the contraction of a muscle. Alexander had stumbled onto a remarkable skill he later termed inhibition. This was an appropriate choice. By telling himself not to speak, he learned to prevent the neural activity that triggered his unwanted physical behavior.*

This was a welcome success, but there was still a problem. He had not yet succeeded in speaking, only in inhibiting the muscle tension that was triggered when he thought of speaking. In time Alexander learned that his first task was to inhibit his thought of speaking, since this restored a more normal way of moving his head and neck. Then the challenge was to speak—but without disturbing this new and better use of his body. To do this he acquired another skill that he later termed *directing*. Alexander gave himself specific verbal instructions that described this new and better pattern of movement: he thought of letting his neck lengthen, letting his head move *forward and up* on his neck, letting his torso *lengthen and widen*, and letting his knees release *forward* from his torso.

Using these new thinking skills, Alexander found that he could prevent his old tension habit and maintain the new coordination of his head and neck as he spoke. While speaking in this way felt

---

* *Inhibition* is often used synonymously with repression, connoting a tendency to hold something in or keep something back, especially an emotion, in a way that is psychologically or physically harmful. By contrast, Alexander's use of the word refers to the positive and healthful capacity of the individual to stop or prevent an unnecessary or harmful behavior.

strange to him, there was no denying the change he saw in the mirror and the improvement he heard in his voice.

At the time Alexander had no idea how *inhibiting* and *directing* produced such remarkable changes. Years later, he drew from the research of a scientist named Rudolf Magnus to formulate a theory. Magnus's work showed that vertebrates have an array of reflexes designed to assist in coordinating the animal's posture and movement that are triggered by the changing position of the head on the neck, and the head's position in relation to gravity. In Magnus's words, in vertebrates "the head leads and the body follows." [1]

Alexander's self-experiments demonstrated the practical side of this research. His misuse of his head and neck was interfering—not just with his voice but with physiological mechanisms designed to assist in coordinating his movements. This in turn marred the overall functioning of his body. By inhibiting, he prevented this misuse. By directing, he maintained the new relationship of his head, neck, and spine as he spoke and as he moved in all his activities. Later, Alexander termed this a **primary control** in the use of himself. In time he noticed that his self-perception shifted as well. The new way of moving felt right to him, and the old way felt wrong. In some unknown way, his mind's interpretation of bodily sensations had become more correct.

Alexander returned to the stage amid wide acclaim. Special compliments were paid to his vocal skill. Then he began to notice that many other people had similar patterns of misuse of themselves, and he began teaching others what he had discovered. Soon his students were reporting significant improvement in a wide array of symptoms, which impressed their physicians. In 1904 Alexander moved to London carrying letters of recommendation from several Australian doctors who admired his work. In a short period, he was teaching his new method to leading figures of the London stage, wealthy patients of respected London physicians, and members of the upper echelons of British society.[2] Alexander relinquished his dream of becoming an actor and devoted himself to teaching his method, which later in his life he described as *the study of human reaction*.

III.

Introduction to the Self-Experiments

The voyage of discovery is not in seeking new landscapes but in having new eyes.
—MARCEL PROUST

L IKE MANY WHO have made important scientific discoveries, Alexander was a keen observer. Then he devised experiments to uncover the meaning of his observations. The subject of study was himself. By observing his body in motion he uncovered his mind in action, as his thoughts played themselves out across the canvas of his body. Through this he gained important insight into the problem of mind-body disconnection: how the mind misinterprets the feelings from the body so that the body often cannot perform even simple movements as the mind intends. In short, we often misjudge ourselves and cannot reliably control what we do. Simple acts done repeatedly, such as slumping in a chair or hunching our shoulders as we hold a pen, feel right to us, and we fail to understand the harm that such simple acts of malcoordination can cause. Further, changing how we move feels wrong, and so we unwittingly perpetuate our mind-body disconnection.

The Alexander Technique is an objective system of self-study that helps us learn to perceive ourselves more accurately. It is a hands-on method that gives us an experience of improved mind-body connection, and that teaches us the tools for change and self-mastery.

How You Stand, How You Move, How You Live is not a substitute for this hands-on learning experience, but if Alexander was able to learn so much through self-observation and experimentation, so, too, can you. Toward that end, the book includes a series of self-experiments that are designed to let you explore your mind-body connection in action, and to learn the central cognitive skills of the method: specifically, sections C and D are designed to teach you how to inhibit; and sections E and F are designed to teach you how to direct. I have developed these procedures over the course of my many years of practice and study of the Technique. While inhibiting and directing were identified and described by Alexander, the self-experiments that explore these essential skills are my own.

Following is a brief overview of the entire series of self-experiments.

Section A teaches you how to rest your back muscles effectively by lying down in the semisupine position (on your back with your hips and knees bent) and in the prone position (face down with your legs straight). In section B, you will observe yourself in movement, specifically as you sit down on and stand up from a chair. You will discover which muscles you use and whether you are tightening your muscles unnecessarily, and you will learn to test your ability to prevent unnecessary tension.

In section C, you will enter the realm of the mind as you begin to learn the most essential skill of the Alexander Technique—conscious inhibition. This section discusses what I term the four pitfalls of learning to inhibit: mind wandering, feeling instead of thinking, thinking mindlessly, and forgetting the meaning of "no." It includes specific steps for learning to recognize and overcome each of these pitfalls. Next, you will combine your skills to practice conscious inhibition. In section D, you will inhibit as you perform a simple movement and experience firsthand how this enables you to prevent unconscious habits of unnecessary tension.

The second skill of the Alexander Technique is directing. Section E begins with experiments designed to help you learn to think spatially and to think in specific spatial directions. Next, you will put these skills together as you practice the directions as Alexander taught them. In section F, you will inhibit and direct as you perform more complex movements, such as moving forward and backward in a chair and progress to standing and sitting. You will experience firsthand how inhibiting prevents unconscious habits that interfere with the optimal functioning of your locomotor system, and how directing enables you to improve your balance and coordination as you move.

In section G, you will practice two simple movements designed to strengthen the deep muscles of your neck and back, the essential muscles of upright posture. Finally, in section H, you will learn how inhibiting and directing can help you exercise and play a sport, overcome performance anxiety, manage chronic pain, and assist you in many of the acts of day-to-day living.

As you explore and practice these self-experiments, keep in mind that your aim is not to achieve a state of perfection but to enjoy a process of self-exploration and discovery. I have termed these "experiments" to encourage you to approach them with curiosity, with openness to new experience, and without fear of failure. Other essential ingredients for success are patience and repetition. In time you will experience the satisfaction and confidence that comes from acquiring new skills and deepening your self-knowledge. Through these self-experiments, you will be following in Alexander's footsteps as you embark on a journey for restoring your mind-body connection to enhance how you live.

HOW DO YOU MOVE?

TALES FROM THE BEGINNING

Surprising Observations

The most erroneous stories are those we think we know best—
and therefore never scrutinize or question.
—STEPHEN JAY GOULD

JOHN, PART ONE

THE DOORBELL RINGS. I pull open the heavy front door
with a twinge of anxiety, which I always feel when meeting a
new student. Today, he is a middle-aged man named John. He
smiles in greeting and I welcome him into the house while taking in a stream of impressions. I watch how he holds his body. I
note the expression on his face, the mood in his eyes, and the timbre of his voice. At this moment of introduction I am like a
prospector hunting for gold, seeking nuggets of detail. I want to
know how he feels inside his skin and how he interprets the
world around him.

As John walks ahead of me into my teaching room, I notice a
quality of heaviness. Despite his slim frame, it appears as if he is carrying an invisible pack, heavily loaded, pressing downward on his
body. He has informed me previously on the phone that he hopes
the Alexander Technique will rid him of the pain he experiences,
day and night, from his frozen right shoulder. Considering his
complaint, John's manner of moving does not surprise me. His

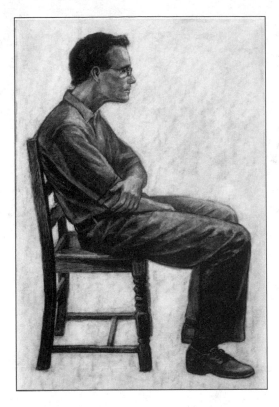

1-1. John sitting collapsed against the back of the chair, neck jutting forward and head pulled back and down on the neck, shoulders rounded forward.

arms are held stiffly against his body, restrained like errant children. One shoulder is lower than the other. His legs barely bend. He lurches his torso from side to side as he walks, pulling each leg up and hoisting it forward.

I invite John to sit down. When he reaches the chair he turns around to face me, pulls his torso forward like a pill bug curling around itself, jerks his head back on his neck, and falls into the chair. My chair creaks as he lands. He finishes the task by collapsing his torso against the back of the chair and, clasping his right elbow with his left hand, sighs audibly (Illustration 1-1). Then he looks past me with a noncommittal expression and says, "Well, I really don't know what you can do for me."

"Tell me what you have already tried for your shoulder, John."

"My doctor sent me to a physical therapist. She gave me some exercises and stretches. I did them for a while but it didn't help."

"Anything else?"

"I've had some massage, which feels good, but it doesn't really change anything. My shoulder still hurts. I can't lift my elbow more than a few inches." He puts his left hand on his right shoulder, squeezes it, and slowly circles his arm to demonstrate its limited range of motion. As he does this, his facial muscles tense from discomfort.

"Anything else?"

"No. I probably have to learn to live with it."

"Everyone is different, but from my experience I'd say it's likely the Alexander Technique can help you. Let me begin by asking you to stand in front of the chair."

As I observe John standing, I see the effect of decades-old contraction. His upper back rounds forward. Since his neck is curved forward as well, his head pulls back on his neck so that he can see out in front of him. His knees are locked. His pelvis is thrust forward.

"Would you sit down once and stand up again? I want to watch what you do."

As John begins to sit, the curve in his spine increases as if a downward push is necessary to make his legs bend. When he reaches the chair, he begins his upward return with the same curling movement in his spine. When he finishes, his torso does not extend upward to its full length but remains in its partial curl, his head positioned back on his neck. John's arms are still pressed inward against his ribs.

"John, let me ask you a question. Do you know what you are doing in your upper back, and your head and neck as you move?"

John's face is blank. "I have no idea," he answers.

"Let's try an experiment. Stand and sit again, but this time see what you can notice happening with your head and neck as you move."

John nods, then sits and stands again. As he finishes he turns to look at me but doesn't speak.

"What did you notice? Anything come to your attention?"

"Not really."

"You didn't move your head and neck at all?"

"Not really. No, I don't think so."

"Let's do a slightly different experiment. This time I'd like you to put your hand on the back of your neck and head. Don't press hard; gently feel what's happening in your body as you move."

John's gaze drops down as he does as I have instructed. When he finishes, he doesn't speak.

"Notice anything?" I ask. "Don't worry, this isn't a test. You can't fail. Tell me whatever you notice."

"Well, it felt as if the muscles in my neck were working. They're tightening, I guess." He pauses. "I didn't know they were doing that."

"Yes, that's it. You felt that with your hand, right? What about your head? Could you feel what it was doing?"

Without comment, John sits and stands again, hand in place, engaged more fully now in the process of self-observation. "Well, it seems to move."

"Which way?"

"Sort of backward, toward the back of my neck. I guess my neck muscles are tightening and pulling my head backward."

"That's right. Can you feel what happens to your neck as a result?" John sits down and stands up but remains silent, thinking about what to say next.

"I guess the muscles in my neck are tensing, pulling my head back, which makes my neck jut forward. The back of my head gets closer to my shoulders."

"That's good. You've described it well. By putting your hand on yourself to feel, you have more information about what you are doing. The first time you tried it, you said nothing was happening, remember? Now you have a different idea about it. Is that a fair statement?"

John smiles, nodding. "Yeah, I had no idea I did this."

"You're not alone. This is what Alexander observed himself doing. Most people do this. It's just a matter of varying degrees. And, like Alexander, most people don't know they're doing it. It is kind of surprising, when you think about it. It's our body and we're the ones making it do what it does, yet there's a lot we don't notice about how we use it. Ready for another experiment?"

"Okay."

"This time leave your hand on your neck to feel what's happening, but see if you can sit and stand without tensing the muscles in your neck and pulling your head back. At this point we don't know whether this is necessary, we only know that you do it. Experiment and see if you can stop doing it."

John puts his hand on his neck again and begins to sit down. This time he moves more slowly and his body looks stiff as he tries to prevent his neck and head from moving. With effort he reaches the chair, but his head and neck have done the same thing as before. "What did you notice?" I ask.

"I think I got tense all over. And my neck still tightened."

"That's right. You tried a common strategy. It's as if we think we can prevent ourselves from tensing one muscle by tensing all the others. That's not a great solution. It makes moving much more difficult. It's like tying your ankles together and trying to run a race. Any other ideas?"

John puts his hand on his neck again and begins to stand up, pivoting his body slowly forward from his hips. This time his neck is lengthening and his head has not pulled back. Then he stops. Just as he begins to increase the tension in his leg muscles to stand, the tension in his neck suddenly reasserts itself. John notices this and, not commenting, sits down. Again he pivots his body slowly forward, stops, and then starts to stand, but he tenses his neck muscles again as he begins to use his legs. Silent, he tries once more. The same responses are triggered. John sits back in the chair and looks at me. "It's not possible," he says, shaking his head. "I can't sit or stand without tensing my neck and pulling my head back! Maybe it has to be like that?"

"This is good, John. You're making important discoveries. You're learning that you have a particular way of using your body. Until now you weren't aware of this. Becoming more aware is the first step, but it isn't sufficient for change. That's what these lessons will teach you how to do."

"Maybe it isn't possible," John says under his breath.

"Okay, that's a fair point. Why don't you watch me sit and stand. Tell me what you observe." After I finish, I turn to him. "Well?"

"You didn't tense your neck or pull your head back at all!"

"Right. So we've answered that question. You don't have to do it. This is your habit. It's part of your particular way of moving your body. Most people create lots of unnecessary tension as they move but they don't feel it, and so they don't realize it's happening.

"What do you think these discoveries might help us learn about this right shoulder that's giving you trouble?"

"Oh that," John says quickly with a tone of relief. "I know what I do there. I know I make it worse because I pull my right shoulder up around my ear."

"Really?"

"Oh yeah, I know that's a big reason why it hurts."

As a teacher with years of experience, I have an advantage. I know what John is doing with his shoulder and it isn't what he thinks. Instead of telling him this, however, I want to give him an opportunity to make this discovery himself.

"I tell you what, John. Let's do something else. Turn right and face the large mirror on the wall. Take a moment to observe your shoulders. Are they the same?"

"No," John says hesitantly, wrinkling his forehead. "My right shoulder looks a bit lower than my left." The tone in John's voice tells me he is having trouble believing what he is seeing.

"Yes. Earlier you were getting information by using your hand to feel your body's movements. Now you're getting information by observing in the mirror. Let's do another experiment. Lift your arms up in front of you as if you were holding a pen, writing at your desk." John quickly mimes the act of writing.

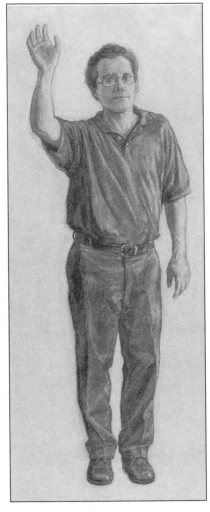

1-2. John standing with right arm raised, right elbow bent, and right shoulder lower than the left, and the left arm held stiffly and pulled back.

"Now look in the mirror. What's your right shoulder doing?"

"It's kind of pushing downward again. It's lower than before."

"Yes. Now watch in the mirror and we'll do another experiment. Lift your left arm over your head, just as far as it can comfortably move, and then bring it down slowly. Watch how you do it. Then, do the same thing with your right arm. Lift it to wherever it's able to go—don't force it—but observe how you move your arm, and especially what happens in your shoulder."

John raises his left arm easily and lowers it. Next he raises his right arm, slowly and more carefully, keeping his elbow bent (Illustration 1-2). Then he brings it down to his side.

"What did you notice? Any difference?"

"Well, my right arm didn't go very far. I knew that would happen. But look at my right shoulder!"

"Yes?"

"My right shoulder is really pressing down. I'm kind of lopsided, now that I look at myself. The whole right side of my torso looks kind of compressed. I look like I'm leaning to the right!"

"From observing yourself doing these movements, would you say that you have a tendency to pull your right shoulder up?"

"No," he says, disbelief rising in his voice. "I don't lift my right shoulder at all. I press it down!"

A Malfunctioning Locomotor System

*All truths are easy to understand once they are discovered;
the point is to discover them.*
—GALILEO GALILEI

ERIN, PART ONE

A SHORT, SLENDER woman in her early forties, Erin is an elementary school teacher. She has come to me complaining of lower back pain, occasional numbness in her left leg, and tingling in her left foot. She has been diagnosed with spinal stenosis, a narrowing of the intervertebral canal in the lower spine, caused by a buildup of calcium deposits pressing on her spinal cord.

Sitting in the chair in my teaching room, Erin describes how this problem is curtailing her activities, especially her ability to play tennis, which, she says with some emotion, is at the heart of her life. Erin looks despondent as she tells me how difficult it is to give this up as her physician has recommended. He has told her that surgery is the only solution but he does not advise it until her symptoms are more severe.

I begin by explaining to Erin that since the Alexander Technique is an educational approach, not a therapeutic one, it is not my role to give her a diagnosis, offer specific treatments, or promise to cure her condition. What I can do is teach her to improve the way that she uses her body in everything she does. In the process she will learn to move with less tension in her muscles, reducing the compression on her spine. In turn this may gradually lessen her symptoms.

"Alexander teachers are in part movement specialists," I explain, keeping the discussion simple. "We teach you about how your body is designed to be used, how you are misusing it, and how you can consciously learn to restore it to better functioning. Your body is a composite of many different systems: respiratory, digestive, reproductive, and so on. Among these is what is commonly called your musculoskeletal system, but I prefer to call it your **locomotor system**. This is a better term, since it describes what it does. It's the system that gives you the ability to move, to do things, and to get from place to place. We all learn to use this system, but how we do it is largely unconscious.

"When we move with too much muscle tension, compressing vertebrae and joints and pulling ourselves out of balance, this system can't function well. It's like driving the car with the emergency brake on. Tension and imbalance put stress and strain on your muscles, joints, bones, and nerves. It restricts your breathing, interferes with circulation, and more. Over time this can lead to all sorts of problems.

"Through the Alexander Technique you can learn to use your locomotor system more efficiently and skillfully. In the process many people experience significant improvement in a wide array of symptoms, including those such as yours."

"What about exercise?" Erin asks.

"Exercise doesn't teach you to change the way that you move. Since how you move is unconscious, you will simply reinforce this way of moving as you exercise. Further, exercises that are designed to strengthen specific muscles may do more harm than good. Since many problems are caused from too much tension, exercises that are designed to increase muscle strength can make the problem worse. Often we need to do less work in our muscles, not more. In addition, exercising a few specific muscles is not the same thing as learning to coordinate your whole body efficiently in everything you do: walking and climbing stairs, brushing your hair, driving the car, or mowing the lawn."

Erin is sitting in front of me. As we talk I observe her closely. She does not look comfortable. There is barely any movement in her ribs as she breathes. Her thighs are pressed together and her heels are pulled up off the floor. Her shoulders are hunched inward. Her fingers rest oddly in her lap, stiffly curled. She is a picture of tension (Illustration 2-1).

"Now, to begin, Erin, would you stand up from the chair and then sit back down again? Let me watch how you move."

As Erin starts to stand, the tension I already noticed becomes more pronounced. Her knees pull more inward, her fingers clench. She tips her pelvis forward, increasing the curve in her lower back. Her neck flattens and she tenses her jaw. As she straightens her legs she also clutches her back muscles, compressing her spine. She stands with obvious pain (Illustration 2-2).

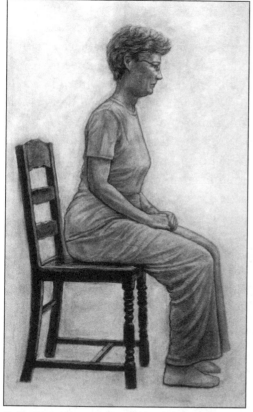

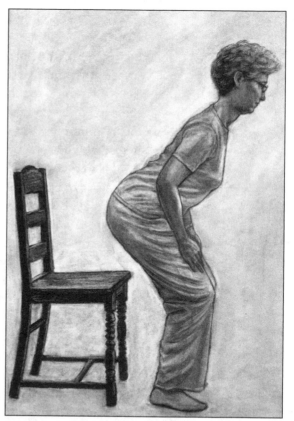

2-1. Erin sitting with neck stiff and flattened, jaw pulled back, shoulders squeezed together and raised, and pelvis tilted forward with the lower back arched, knees squeezed together.

2-2. Erin starting to stand, tipping the pelvis forward with excessive tightening in muscles at the front of the hips as the back muscles tighten and pull the chest backward, unduly flattening the upper spine. The knees are squeezed together and the arms are bent at the elbows with fingers curled.

Next Erin begins to sit down. First her pelvis tips forward. This pulls her body forward onto the balls of her feet. Then she tenses even more in her legs to prevent herself from falling. This means that she is tightening just the muscles that must lengthen in order to allow her joints to bend. Erin is literally preventing herself from sitting with too much muscle tension, then tensing her muscles even more to overcome this self-imposed resistance. Then suddenly she relaxes everything and falls into the chair. She positions her body as before, tilts her head, and shrugs her shoulders as if to say, "I'm doing my best. What more can I do?"

AT FIRST GLANCE John's and Erin's complaints seem unrelated. Not surprisingly, they have received different diagnoses and treatments. What could pain and stiffness in the shoulder have in common with numbness in the leg and back pain? But if we focus on their symptoms and assume that their problems begin and end in the part of the body that hurts, we will fail to see that they have a lot in common. Erin and John are seriously misusing their locomotor systems. The only true solution for eradicating their symptoms is to restore this system to normal functioning: Erin and John must learn to prevent the movement habits that are seriously pulling their bodies out of kilter, and learn to move their bodies more consciously with efficiency and skill.

To better understand what this means, in the next two chapters we will take a closer look at **bipedalism**, the human locomotor strategy of carrying the torso vertically on top of two straightened and weight-bearing hind limbs. We will consider how humans evolved to be upright and how every human child learns to stand. We will explore the unique demands of our locomotor strategy, and learn to better appreciate its advantages while more fully understanding its perils. In short, we will discover why we are beautifully designed for standing upright and moving with balance and coordination but too often fail to achieve it.

How Did We Get This Way?

From Fish to Horse to Biped

> You cannot teach a crab to walk straight.
> —ARISTOPHANES

ALL ANIMALS POSSESS their own means of transportation—a personal horse and buggy. The single-celled paramecium moves across its aqueous environment with a flick of its cilia-tail. Other animals have devised more complex locomotor strategies. They have acquired muscles, bones, joints, neurons, and specialized areas of the brain to enable them to move individual parts as well as the whole of themselves, and so to travel from place to place.

The earliest vertebrates lived in a watery world. They acquired a skull to protect their increasingly important brain, and articulating vertebrae to protect the spinal cord while also permitting range of motion. They gained muscles that spanned the length of this vertebral column and nerves to innervate them, generating rhythmically alternating contractions to bend the body laterally, first on one side and then the other. This sideward bending was not random but precisely coordinated. *It functioned to orient and propel the animal in the direction of its head*—site of eyes, nose, mouth, teeth, and increasingly complex brain. In this first or *primary* vertebrate locomotor system, *the animal's body followed its head's direction.*

The first amphibians and later the reptiles moved out of the water by turning gills into lungs and fins into emerging limbs. Other locomotor strategies were derived as offshoots of this. Birds turned scales into feathers and forelimbs into wings to leave the ground altogether.

Eventually this limbed creature made further changes, becoming a mammal and a true **quadruped**, with four appendages made of long, strong bones. These supported the animal's trunk upward from below, carrying the body up off the ground. Additional, larger muscles were required to move these limbs, support the body's weight, and stabilize the trunk as it moved. Rather than entirely revamping the primary locomotor system, nature layered new muscles on top of those that came before, configuring them in a sort of double helix arrangement that wrapped around the trunk and spiraled downward onto the limbs.[1]

The quadruped's chief means of propulsion was no longer a laterally bending spine leveraging itself against the water's resistance, but four limbs moving in coordinated synchrony, feet pushing against the ground to propel the animal forward—not through water but air. *The quadruped's chief direction of movement was still toward its head, but now a second orienting direction became important: toward the earth and gravity's pull.* With every weight-bearing step, the musculature of each limb coordinated its movement toward the ground. It was this leveraging, pushing action against the earth that provided the animal its means of propulsion. The many mechanisms and structures that evolved to make this quadrupedal locomotor strategy possible constitute what I term a *secondary* locomotor system.

Some quadrupeds moved up into the trees to become **brachiators**. Now the muscles in the upper body and forelimbs became more powerful, enabling the animal to suspend its body from overhead branches and travel by swinging from one to the next. The forelimbs became adapted to this new environment with articulating hands and fingers for grasping, and forearms that rotated.

Some scientists theorize it was these brachiators who occasionally fell out of the trees and then remained increasingly on the ground, acquiring greater strength in the muscles of the hind limbs to become **semibrachiators**. These animals retained the brachiator's adaptations in the forelimbs, but used their stronger hind limbs to support their body, while the knuckles of the hands were used to bear weight as the animal traveled.

Next some of these semibrachiators acquired another locomotor strategy. Their torso pivoted backward from the hip joints, positioning the head and spine vertically on top of two increasingly straight hind legs, the arms no longer weight-bearing but swinging freely in counterbalance with the hind limbs, the hands already adapted for carrying and holding. *Now a third direction of orientation became important—up—the direction opposite to gravity.* These fully upright bipeds left the forest behind and strode out across the savannah. Bipedalism, a uniquely human means of locomotion was born (Illustration 3-1).

This human locomotor strategy, which embodies many of the central features of the fish and the quadruped, also depends on a distinctly new capacity. Standing on two feet is a delicately adjusting and readjusting balancing act. When we walk, this balancing function becomes even more critical as we step onto each successive forward limb, head and torso poised over the front leg as the foot behind pushes against the ground to propel us forward. We no longer actively move in the direction of our head (as the fish and quadruped do), but toward the front of our body. It might even be said that our gait is that of a monoped as, continuing to balance, we transfer our entire body from single limb to single limb. And as we run, for brief moments we become limbless again, propelling ourselves into space and leaving the earth (for brief moments) altogether.

Thus we can trace the course of vertebrate evolution through these successive locomotor strategies, from the fish swimming in suspension with its sinewy spine following its head's lead; to the quadrupedal creature still propelling its body toward its head like the

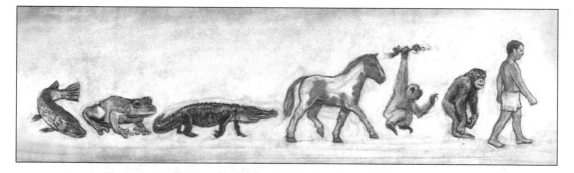

3-1. Evolution of vertebrate locomotor systems: fish, amphibian, reptile, quadruped, brachiator, semibrachiator, and biped.

fish but now extending its weight-bearing, bendable limbs toward the earth to carry its trunk off the ground; to the bipedal human balancing its head and trunk vertically on top of extending legs, the arms and hands adapted to shape its environment to its intent.

We see a similar progression repeated within each of us as we grow. Every human begins life in the womb as a fishlike embryo. The newborn infant lies on its belly, horizontal to the ground, beginning its journey toward bipedalism by lifting its head off the ground to see the world and developing the strength of its back muscles. (You will try this movement in the self-experiments in section G.) After several months the baby begins extending its arms to push its upper torso off the ground. Eventually it gains sufficient strength to push its trunk to a vertical position, plant its bottom on the floor, and balance its torso upright while sitting. At about seven months the baby progresses from sitting to crawling on its hands and knees—a brief stint as a quadruped—before becoming the beaming-faced toddler that, imitating its elders, maintains its vertically balancing head and trunk while straightening its legs and then, teetering precariously at first, takes its first steps (Illustration 3-2). Each human's upright stance is achieved, not over the span of millennia, but over a nine-month gestation plus a year beyond birth.

Let us look a little more closely at how you stand.

When your torso is upright the deepest muscles of your back that are located close to your vertebrae—the muscles of your primary locomotor system—support your head and spinal column with ease. These deep muscles are *involuntary*. You cannot contract them consciously or feel them working, but a six-month-old coordinates their action sufficiently to balance its torso vertically while sup-

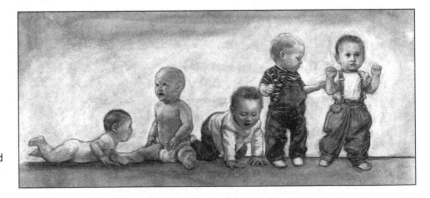

3-2. Progression of human infant locomotor development: lying belly down with head and upper body lifted; sitting with torso balanced vertically and head poised on top of spine; crawling; standing; walking.

porting its heavy head. (Babies fall over easily at this stage, because if the head moves too far away from its axis of support there is not yet sufficient strength in the larger, more superficial muscles of the trunk to counter its weight.)

Your head is poised on top of your spine but—and this is important—its center of gravity is slightly in front of the spine, not directly above it. In addition, the head's center of gravity is in front of the center of gravity of the torso. This arrangement puts a slight stretch on the muscles at the back of the neck and spine, increasing their tonus (a normal muscle's state of partial contraction) to help support the head's weight. In addition, the muscles of the back are inherently stronger than the muscles in the front of the body. (A baby lying on its stomach can lift its head with the muscles at the back of the head and neck not long after birth, but a child is closer to five years old before it can lie on its back and lift its head with the muscles in the front of the neck.) This arrangement also means that the full weight of the head is not pressing directly downward onto the spine. This helps to prevent both undue compression of disks and harmful distortion of normal spinal curvatures.

The strong, supple spinal column is not straight but gently curved, giving it greater tensile strength to help support your head from below. Your twelve pairs of ribs are jointed to the twelve chest or thoracic vertebrae. Breathing is coordinated by the contraction of the diaphragm, and also by the action of the intercostal muscles, located between the ribs, which pull them apart and then together in rhythmic expansion and contraction. As your ribs move, the deep muscles of the back continue to maintain the vertical integrity of your spinal column.

In conjunction with the deep muscles of the spine, the quadrupedal double-spiral arrangement in the outer muscles of the trunk and limbs work to both stabilize the limbs as they are weight-bearing and move them in smooth synchrony for walking, running, jumping, and climbing. Distinct from the deep back muscles, these superficial muscles are *voluntary*—their action is more readily felt and is linked to higher cortical areas of the brain, allowing you greater conscious control of their action.

A central feature differentiating our locomotor strategy from that of the quadruped and even the semibrachiator is the position of the head on the spine. Another is the different position of the head and

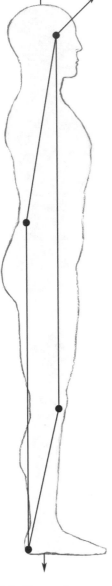

torso relative to the ground. These changes have required further adaptations. Although we appear to stand vertically—our head on top of a vertical spine on top of two straight legs—as we have seen, the head's center of gravity and the centers of gravity of the torso and the legs are not positioned directly over one another but are slightly skewed. This creates an inherently unstable relationship between our many jointed parts: Our mobile head rests on top of a mobile and jointed vertebral column. The moveable trunk rests on top of bendable legs. The centers of gravity of the legs are not directly beneath the torso's center of gravity but slightly in front of it. Further, our spinal column is not positioned in the center of our torso (as we might expect of a creature whose trunk is aligned in the same vertical direction as it legs) but in the back of our torso, behind our central axis.

Your upright stance, then, is not achieved through a system of static alignment. Your bones are not straight. Your chief centers of weight are not lined up, one on top of the other, like a stack of carefully placed building blocks. Your head's center of gravity is forward and up from your spine, your trunk's center of gravity is back and down relative to your head. Your legs are not bent as you stand but straight, yet their center of gravity is slightly in front of the torso. Finally, your heels extend back from your ankles, away from the legs, back and down into the ground (Illustration 3-3).

As a result of these slightly skewed centers of gravity, it is the deep muscles of your back that are chiefly responsible for maintaining the upright poise of your head and trunk. And it is the muscles at the back of your hips, the front of your knees, and the back of your ankles and bottoms of your feet that do the small amount of work necessary to keep your legs straight as you stand. (Thus, standing on two feet requires the use of the *extensor* muscles, not the *flexor* muscles.)

Ours is a system not of static balance but of *dynamic counterbalance.* Our slightly opposing centers of weight (head, torso, legs, and heels) exert a steady stimulus of gentle, oppositional stretch on our muscles, slightly increasing their tonus. This means that our body maintains its uprightness not through a system of tight, shortened, bulky musculature that grips mightily to hold us in place, but rather through a system of supple and lengthening musculature that supports us in our vertical stance with a minimum of effort while allowing mobility. Ours is an exquisite design that maintains our balance

3-3. Human figure, profile view: schema showing approximate placement of centers of gravity of head, trunk, and legs.

as we walk upright with little effort and little compression on our joints. As bipeds we are designed to move with balance, coordination, and near effortlessness.

Frequently cited advantages of our uprightness include our muscular endurance that enables us to travel long distances; the elevation of our eyes to see out across the horizon; the freedom of our hands to hold and manipulate objects; and the reduction in total body surface that is directly exposed to the sun. What is often overlooked is that this dynamically counterbalancing system is remarkably efficient. It requires significantly less muscular work to stand via our system of dynamic counterbalance than, for example, the work that is required of a semibrachiator. Bipedalism was a distinct advantage for our early forbears. Since it requires less muscle strength, it requires less muscle mass.[2] Less muscle mass means lowered dietary needs. Times of limited food supply would be less critical. And any surplus calories could be used to feed other bodily structures, such as an increasingly large and nutrient-hungry brain.

Contrary to what many people believe, we are exquisitely adapted for our uprightness. Many structural and neurological changes took place to progress from the semibrachiator to the upright stance. The spinal curvatures in the neck and lower back increased; there were changes in the shape of pelvic and leg bones; our ribcage became wider and shallower, shifting the center of gravity of the torso backward; the site of attachment of the skull on the spine moved forward. The **vestibular apparatus** in the inner ear became increasingly important for spatial orientation and balance. (More on this in part 4.) Sensory receptors throughout the body increased to give the brain vital information about the body's position and movements in space, helping it to monitor and maintain the body's delicately counterbalancing uprightness. We could characterize these and many more such changes as constituting a *third* vertebrate locomotor system.

Thus, like a layer cake, we are many-tiered. Our locomotor system has been built upon the systems that

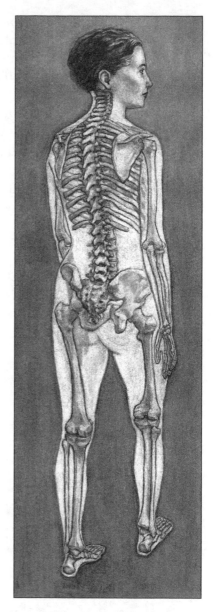

3-4. Walking skeleton with good alignment: the neck is slightly curved and lengthening upward; the head is poised forward and up on top of the spine; the shoulder blades are spreading wide across the back; the spine is gently curved; the head is aligned over the pelvis; the body's weight is correctly distributed over the feet.

have come before. We are each an elegant blend of fish, horse, and upwardly lengthening, efficiently counterbalancing biped (see Illustration 3-4).

But if we are so well adapted for standing upright, why are we so often in pain, out of balance and hunched over, stressed out, and unable to relax? Why do we suffer so much wear and tear? Why do so many of us complain that moving our body and standing upright is difficult, uncomfortable, fatiguing? What causes the many musculoskeletal complaints that have reached near-epidemic proportions in modern humans? As we will see in the next chapter, while bipedalism has its advantages, it presents some distinct challenges.

Standing on Two Legs

The Biped's Challenge

We first make our habits, and then they make us.
—JOHN DRYDEN

THE PICTURE I have painted thus far of how we stand is incomplete. Bipedalism requires another highly specialized system: our capacity to learn. We do not walk because it is an instinct, hardwired within us, operating infallibly with clockwork precision. We walk because we learn to do it.[1]

This learning demands not only a larger brain but also a more flexible and adaptable brain, a brain that can receive and integrate vast amounts of sensory input and make rapid, subtle adjustments and readjustments that enable us to maintain our upright poise as we move. Ours is a brain that can feel, assess, judge, and synthesize what is happening in each part, as well as be aware of the whole, override a misstep, remember how we performed a previous action, plan our next move, decide where we will go, and continually learn new skills. Living upright is for us quite literally a balancing act, one that must be learned and sustained as we perform our activities. To be more precise, we should call this our *psycholocomotor system.*

In contrast to humans, squirrels running across the branch outside my window all look and move the same. It is hard to distinguish them one from the other by their gait. They do not learn to use their locomotor system as we do; it is more hardwired. And since they do not learn to use it, they also do not learn to *misuse* it.

Although our uprightness is learned, this is largely a subconscious process. Through unconscious imitation and trial and error, we learn to perform virtually every movement we make—standing, walking, running, speaking, writing, peeling carrots, even reading. This learning means that, while we are all bipeds, in practical terms we each invent our own unique variation, creating a one-of-a-kind locomotor strategy. Watch people walking down the street. Do they move the same? Have you noticed that you can distinguish a friend walking in front of you by a characteristic hunch in the shoulders or a familiar sway of the hips? Consider how unique each person's handwriting is.

Not only is our uprightness learned, it must be sustained. It isn't a fixed position or posture that we can achieve, lock ourselves into, and then ignore as we turn our mind to other matters. Our uprightness must be continually renewed and restored as we travel through space, as we move just a part of our body, and even as we are upright but unmoving. This counterbalancing system is fragile, affected merely by the movement of our ribs as we breathe.

We might readily ask why anyone would think of putting a heavy, ten- to twelve-pound head on top of a long, thin spinal column and then move about by shifting this top-heavy column from single foot to single foot? With the slightest misstep our finely tuned counterbalance is thrown askew. We risk tumbling to the ground and causing injury or must grip our muscles in sudden contraction to prevent a fall. Every clutch of our musculature to prevent such catastrophe applies a sudden compression force on our structure. Yet we have little awareness of the strain and tension growing within us, moment by moment, year after year. After decades of contraction and downward pressure, the majority of us suffer from a wide array of musculoskeletal pains and complaints.

Perhaps now we can frame a better picture in our mind of our very human contradictions. The primary locomotor system within us—the fish—should be supporting our supple spine, sustaining our trunk in its lengthening, toward-the-head orientation, but instead we collapse downward, compressing this structure. Our secondary locomotor system—the quadruped—should be rhythmically coordinating our limbs away from our trunk and orienting them toward the ground, but instead we hold them retracted stiffly inward against our body. Our third locomotor system—the exquisitely counterbalancing biped—should continually adjust and readjust itself in counterbalance to maintain the body's uprightness, but instead we grip too hard, clutching our muscles to keep from falling, overriding this balancing system (Illustration 4-1).

To see this in action, let us return to John and Erin. With a more knowledgeable eye, we have good reason for alarm, not only because of their specific complaints but also because of the stark evidence of decline in the use and functioning of their psycholocomotor systems. John's walk resembles the shuffling of stiffened tree limbs. His arms are pulled in and forward, causing downward pressure on his torso. His legs barely move. His spine is seriously collapsed, causing severe strain on muscles, disks, joints, and nerves, and impeding his respiratory functioning. He does not perceive this, however, and does not understand that he is literally wearing out his body from unconscious misuse. Instead, John believes all is well—except for that annoying right shoulder (see Illustration 4-2).

At first glance Erin's torso appears to be more upright, but on closer examination we see its stiffness. Like John's, Erin's arms are taut and pulled into her torso, but unlike his, they are also pulled back, slightly behind her body. Erin barely breathes. The tension in her leg muscles and abdomen is extreme. Due to this tension, sitting down and standing up require tremendous effort, putting excess pressure on her vertebrae, disks, and nerves. Immobilizing tension is spread throughout her body, from her stiffened neck to the tips of her fingers and brief smile. Erin's chief complaint is that

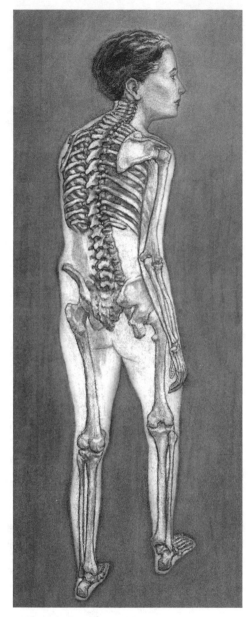

4-1. Walking skeleton with poor alignment: the neck is jutting forward, increasing the neck's curvature; the head is pulled back and down on the spine; the chest is collapsed forward and down; the shoulder blades are pulled forward; the pelvis is tipped back, flattening the normal curvature in the lumbar spine; the body's weight is distributed over the insides of the feet.

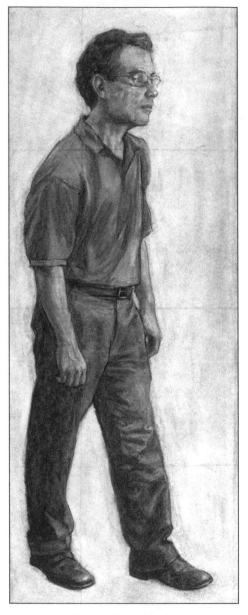

4-2. John walking with neck collapsed forward, head pulled back, and right shoulder and arm pulled down.

she wants to be able to play tennis again, but she does not realize that it is how she plays tennis that is preventing her from playing (Illustration 4-3).

John and Erin are not the exceptions to the rule but the standard. Observe those around you and listen to their complaints: back pain, shoulder pain, knee pain, carpal tunnel syndrome, tennis elbow, jaw pain, foot pain, hip pain, muscle stiffness, tendinitis, arthritis, ruptured disks, shortened muscles that restrict mobility, mind wandering, emotional overreaction, difficulty performing simple tasks such as bending down to lift the laundry basket or getting up from the sofa. Such problems are epidemic. Despite its advantages, our bipedalism comes at a heavy price.

Why is it so difficult? The greatest challenge of uprightness is that it is in large measure a neurological/mental act, not just a simple muscular/physical one. As such, uprightness must be learned and learned well, and skillfully maintained—even as we turn our attention to other tasks. Each of us accomplishes this skill with more or less success. Just as some play the piano better than others, some achieve greater skill in the use of our locomotor system. Subconscious patterns of tension that seriously interfere with our locomotor functioning can be acquired at any time throughout our lives. Injury, illness, fear, emotional stress, long hours of repetitive activity, and cultural norms and pressures all play their part in teaching us (largely below conscious awareness) an array of harmful patterns of tension and ways of moving that disturb our upright balance and impede our overall coordination.

What is more, we do not possess a built-in gauge for accurately judging our tension and malcoordination. A bell does not ring in our heads when we pull ourselves out of balance. Dimly aware of the state of disequilibrium within us, we make vague efforts to right our ills by treating symptoms, or exercising to increase our muscle strength. But medication cannot change the harmful habits that accompany our actions. Lifting weights at the gym does not teach us to skillfully maintain our upright poise. Running a marathon does not prevent us from sitting in a heap all day at our desks. Medications cannot undo the wear and tear of decades of excess pressure on cartilage and joints. Psychotherapy will not fix our anxious gestures and hunching shoulders. Expensive, orthopedically designed desk chairs do not teach us to sit in balance. An expensive week at the spa filled with massages, a low-fat diet, and a tailor-made exercise regimen does not teach us to use our locomotor system skillfully.

We pride ourselves on the vast potential of our conscious mind, yet due to our unconsciously learned habits most of us have far less choice than we believe. We can decide to go for a walk, but cannot decide to walk without our misuse. We can decide to do an exercise, but cannot perceive that we are doing it incorrectly. We do not know what is right, and we do not know how to change. We have left the attainment of our locomotor skill to chance and circumstance. Failing to master our uprightness, bipeds are possibly evolution's sorriest example— creatures that unwittingly create their own self-imposed ills and then must bear the brunt of their oversight.

Ironically, it is also the demands of balance

4-3. Erin walking with neck flattened back, jaw pulled back, head forward and down, shoulders pulled back and lifted, elbows bent and fingers curled, lower back too arched and the upper back unduly flattened.

and uprightness that over the millennia have played a large part in developing our brain's *plasticity*, our enormous capacity to change and learn. Ours is the brain that learns to play a Paganini violin concerto, to climb a mountain, to build a skyscraper. Ours is the brain that produces the jumps of Michael Jordan and the leaps of Baryshnikov. We are exceptionally adaptable: we can learn, unlearn, and relearn throughout our lifetime. It is our blend of unconscious, reflexive locomotor systems (the fish and the quadruped) combined with our vast capacity for learning (the biped) that enables us to climb ever higher in accomplishment and achievement. As far as we know, only bipeds possess this new order of mind, a mind capable of self-awareness, self-direction, and self-learning—that is to say, a mind that is highly *self-intelligent*.

But we must not proclaim our talents too quickly. How many of us become Michael Jordan? Yo-Yo Ma? Renée Fleming? Tiger Woods? Their successes are the exception, not the norm. We take collective pride in the remarkable achievements of members of our species, but few of us attain a high level of skill in the use of our organism. Why does an animal made for self-mastery so seldom achieve it? Why do so few of us fulfill the biped's promise?

It is tempting to put the blame on the rigors of daily existence: sitting in chairs, staring at computer screens, long years in school. But it is not in the stress and demands of civilized life that we find the chief cause of our dilemma. The clue to the puzzle lies in paradox. As bipeds we are caught in evolution's march. We straddle a divide. We stand between earlier, unconscious mechanisms of control that precisely govern movement and behavior but permit little learning, and our evolving capacity for self-awareness and consciousness that give us vast potential to learn but do not govern *how* we learn.

In sum, the chief source of our difficulty lies in our biology. We learn, but we learn imperfectly and incorrectly. What is more, a creature that makes mistakes needs to be able to self-correct. But self-correction depends on accurate self-judgment, and we seldom perceive ourselves accurately. Our brain is easily tricked and misled. We fail to accurately perceive or fully understand our misuse and our misperceptions. This is perhaps our greatest shortcoming.

In part 2, we will learn that the source of this problem lies in what I call our sixth sense—our brain's sensory system for perceiving and judging what is happening within us. But first we will pause for a series of self-experiments. First you will learn how to rest your back muscles effectively in order to recover from the demands of uprightness. Next you will begin to explore your unconscious use of your locomotor system, and the way that you perceive yourself.

A and B

The more experiments you make the better.
—RALPH WALDO EMERSON

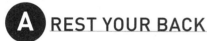 REST YOUR BACK

Take rest; a field that has rested
gives a bountiful crop.
—OVID

As YOU STAND and sit, the small, deep muscles of your back are designed to support your head and torso upright with ease. In contrast, the large, superficial muscles of your back are intended to help you perform larger movements, and tasks requiring greater strength. In short, performed skillfully, standing and sitting require little effort. But while these muscles can support your head and torso with ease, they cannot do this for hours and hours. Your muscles fatigue, and when this happens you find yourself sitting in a slump against the back of your chair, leaning on your elbow at your desk, or collapsing downward into your pelvis as you stand. Or you may unconsciously use the superficial back muscles instead to help you remain upright. But these muscles are not made for the sustained work of uprightness. Eventually, this muscular imbalance becomes habitual: the deep muscles become weaker from collapse and nonuse, and the superficial muscles become increasingly tense. In this state of malcoordination you feel increasingly uncomfortable, finding it harder to sit or stand for long periods. You may also suffer more and more from pain and backache.

In order to restore a skilled coordination to your musculature (using the muscles that are meant for the job and not using the muscles that aren't), you must begin by resting your muscles frequently and effectively. Chronic overwork and imbalance is a condition not just of our lives, but also of our musculature. Frequent periods of rest can help alleviate the problem. This is best done by lying down often for short periods, in positions in which your spine is fully supported and well aligned.

The rest positions that best meet these criteria are semisupine (lying on your back with your knees bent) and prone (lying on your front). These are also good positions for recovering from musculoskeletal injuries, especially of the back, neck, shoulders, and legs. They help let muscles release their grip, reduce compression on joints and spinal disks, improve circulation and breathing, and allow the vertebrae to become gently realigned without force or tension. You may also find that these are good sleeping positions (especially lying in semisupine with pillows under your legs), and can help transform a night's sleep into a healthful rest.

SemiSupine

1. Lie down on your back on a padded and firm surface (Illustration A-1-1).

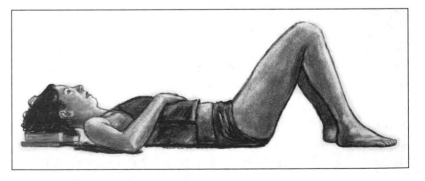

A-1-1. Semisupine: lying on the back on a firm surface, elbows bent with hands on ribs, knees bent, feet placed on the floor a comfortable distance apart. Books are placed under the head to support the head and allow the neck to lengthen without exaggerating or flattening its normal curvature.

Lying on a rug on the floor is best. A bed is all right but a firm surface is better, because it gives your spine more support.

2. **Place several books under your head.**

The books allow your head to be supported as your neck muscles lengthen. If you lie on your back without anything under your head, your neck will either arch too much, causing your head to tilt backward (Illustration A-1-2) or, if you are especially flexible, your neck will flatten too much and lose its normal curvature (Illustration A-1-3). In either case, you are causing compression of the vertebrae and disks in your neck.

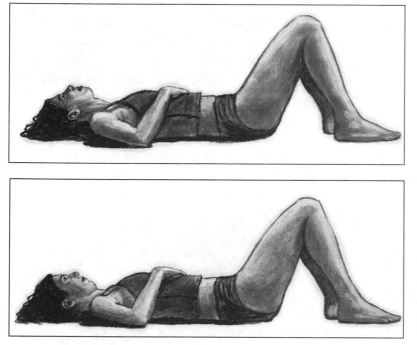

A-1-2. Semisupine, lying on the back with no books under the head: Since the student's neck muscles are tight, the neck curves excessively as the head is pulled back and down on the neck.

A-1-3. Semisupine, lying on the back with no books under the head: Since the student's neck muscles and ligaments are loose, the neck's curvature is eliminated as the jaw presses backward into the throat, and the head is rotated forward and down on the neck.

How many books should you use? Experiment. If there are too many, you will feel your chin pressing uncomfortably against your throat (see Illustration A-1-4). If there are not enough books, you will experience either of the problems described above. Most adults need about two or three inches under the head. If you have a pronounced curvature in your neck or chest, you may need several inches more. If you feel an uncomfortable pressure on the back of your head, fold a

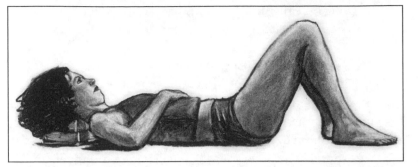

A-1-4. Semisupine: lying on the back with too many books under the head. This causes the mid- and upper-neck curvature to flatten, while the lower neck curves too far forward. It also tends to make the jaw press back, and the head rotate forward and down.

washcloth and place it on top of the books. Do not use a neck pillow. The idea is to support your head, while letting your neck fall slightly back with gravity as it lengthens.

3. Bend your knees, hips, and ankles, and place your feet on the floor. Position your feet a comfortable distance apart, and a comfortable distance from your pelvis.

If your knees have a tendency to fall in or out instead of balancing over your feet, try resting your lower legs on the seat of a chair, or resting your legs on pillows. Use sufficient pillows to support the length of your legs (thighs and calves) so your heels are raised slightly off the floor (Illustration A-1-5).

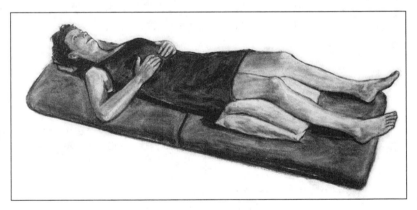

A-1-5. Semisupine: books under the head at optimal height, legs supported by pillows with the hips and knees slightly bent.

4. Bend your arms at your elbows, and rest your hands on your abdomen. Alternatively, you may rest your arms on the floor next to your sides, palms down.

By resting on your back in this position, supported by a firm surface with your head lifted slightly by the books, gravity will gradually exert its gentle pull on your muscles and bones. Muscles will slowly release their grip, and vertebrae will subtly shift and become better aligned.

Do not press your lower back against the floor.
Do not hold in your stomach.
Do not fidget in your body.
Lie still, and simply take time to allow your body to rest.

▶ DISCUSSION

How often should you lie in semisupine and for how long? There is no single answer for everyone, but doing it more often is better. If you can lie down six times a day for ten minutes at a time, this is better than lying down once a day for an hour. Examine your daily routine and environment. Buy an exercise pad and take it to work. Find a quiet, unoccupied space (or shut your office door occasionally) and lie down for five or ten minutes. With the help of gravity and a little patience, your muscles will have a rest as they lengthen. You may be surprised to discover that by doing this several times a day for short periods, aches and pains melt away. You may also notice that when you return to your activities, even after only a few minutes, you are more mentally alert and energized.

Prone

1. Use the books that were under your head in semisupine (or you may use a small pillow) and place them under your chest bone (the sternum) as you lie down on a padded floor, this time with your face down (Illustration A-2-1).

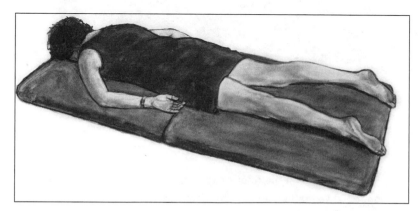

A-2-1. Prone: lying facedown on a firm surface. The arms are placed along the sides of the body with elbows bent and palms up. The shoulders fall forward toward the floor. The backs of the legs face the ceiling with the feet a comfortable distance apart. The head rotates forward on the top of the neck so that it is primarily the forehead rather than the face that contacts the floor.

It is important to use books that are the right size. They should not extend downward beyond your chest bone into your abdominal area. This makes it harder to breathe. They also should not extend too far up toward your head, pressing against your jaw. (*National Geographic* is ideal.)

The purpose of the books is to raise your chest so that your neck falls forward from your back, and your head rotates slightly *forward* on the top of your spine (as if you were nodding "yes"). This allows your upper forehead to rest on the floor rather than your face (Illustration A-2-2). You may require more books than you used in semisupine. If the books are a good height for you, they will prevent your nose from being uncomfortably compressed into the floor (Illustration A-2-3).

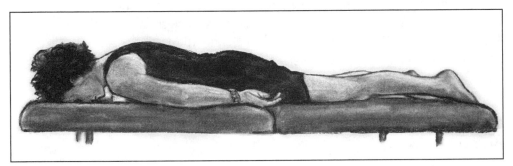

A-2-2. Prone: lying facedown with about three inches of books under the sternum (the bone in the center of the chest) to raise the chest slightly. This helps to allow the neck to lengthen as it falls forward from the upper back, and the head to rotate forward on the neck.

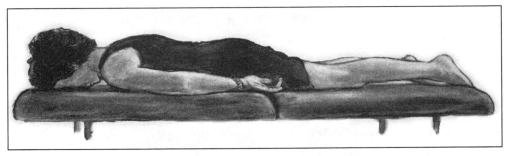

A-2-3. Prone: lying facedown without any books under the chest. Some people have enough flexibility in the neck to do this comfortably. But for most people, lying in prone without anything under the chest causes the nose to press uncomfortably into the floor.

2. Put your arms on the floor next to your sides, palms up, elbows bent. Let your shoulders fall forward, toward the floor.

Do not worry if you feel round-shouldered. Your shoulders will return to their normal position when you are upright.

3. Position your legs so that they are straight, and your feet are several inches apart.

The front surface of your thighs, shins, and tops of your feet should contact the floor. Try not to roll your legs out or in.

4. Let your lower jaw fall slightly open, toward the floor.

The prone position lets the jaw muscles stretch, which is good for jaw pain and tension.

5. Lie in prone for five or ten minutes.

Think about allowing your weight to fall into the floor with gravity. Think of letting go of tension in your back, shoulders, arms, legs, and abdomen. After you become more familiar with this, you can increase the length of time that you rest in prone.

▶ DISCUSSION

Some people like the prone position immediately, while others at first find it uncomfortable and even disconcerting. If you are among the latter, try it for just a few minutes each day until it becomes more comfortable. The main problem with lying in prone for many people is the unusual feeling of pressure on their chest. Experiment with the height of the books until you find what is best for you. You can put a towel or a small pillow on top of the books for cushioning. Do not let this extend down under your abdomen, which would restrict your breathing. The feeling of pressure on your chest can be uncomfortable at first, but put your mind on letting go of your muscles and allowing your body to fall toward the floor. The feeling of pressure usually fades quickly.

Be sure not to hold your breath. If your nose presses uncomfortably into the floor, try using a few more books. If you use too many books, you will feel an increase of pressure on your chest. You must experiment and strike a balance.

Many people are afraid to lie in prone because they have been told that this is bad for their lower back. This is true if you are lying in prone on a sagging mattress, causing an exaggerated curvature in your lower spine. If you are lying on a firm, padded surface, like the one you have used to lie in semisupine, you will be fine.

The prone position has some advantages over semisupine. The most important is that in this position your spine is not weight-bearing. People with chronic low back pain often find that prone gives them more relief from their pain than any other position. It is also helpful for releasing tension in the neck and shoulders.

 ## MOTION AND MIND

> Curious things, habits.
> People themselves never know they have them.
> —AGATHA CHRISTIE

The purpose of these self-experiments is to make observations about how you move. You will become a bit of a scientist, observing and collecting data about how you do what you do. You will probably find that you work some muscles more than necessary, and use others that you do not need. These discoveries can be dismaying, but the first step toward change is becoming aware, so this is progress. Once you become familiar with this process of self-observation, you can apply it to anything you do. As you experiment, remember that your goal is not to try to do the movement correctly but to observe *how* you move.

How You Move

1. Stand in front of a chair. Sit down and stand up several times. What do you notice about how you move?

    Do not worry if at first you do not notice anything. The way you move is habitual. You do not usually think about it. You may find yourself thinking, *Why am I doing this?* This is your mind's way of saying that it is not used to this process of self-observation. Instead of trying to answer the question, remind yourself that your task is simply to observe yourself and gather information.

2. **Sit down and stand up again, this time putting your attention on your head and neck. What do you notice?**

   Again, you may not notice anything. Or you may find yourself thinking, *What am I supposed to notice?* This is your mind asking to be given the answers before you begin, rather than using the process of self-observation to *discover* something new.

3. **Place your hand lightly on the back of your neck and base of your skull. Sit down and stand up several times, using your hand to feel and give you information about what is happening in this area of your body as you move (Illustration B-1-1, B-1-2, B-1-3).**

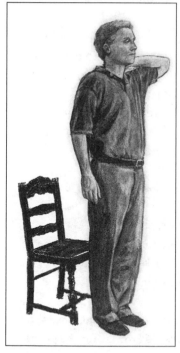

B-1-1. Standing, with hand placed lightly on the back of the neck and head.

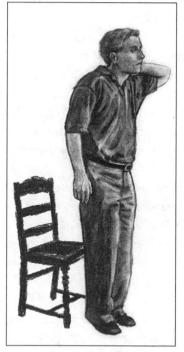

B-1-2. Starting to sit, using the contact of the hand on the back of the head and neck to feel muscle activity and the movement of the head and neck.

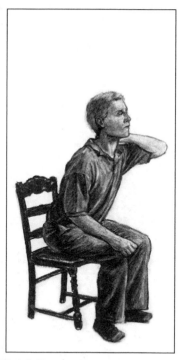

B-1-3. Starting to stand up, using the hand on the head and neck to feel muscle activity and the movement of the head and neck.

Now, you will probably learn more about what you are doing as you move. Your hand helps you feel what your muscles are doing. They may tense and shorten, pulling on the back of your head, moving it back and down onto your neck. You may also feel your neck shifting forward, away from your hand. This means that the curve in your neck is increasing, which increases the compression on the vertebrae and disks in your neck. (See also Illustration II-1.)

Or you may feel yourself doing the opposite movement: Some people tense too much in the muscles in the front of the neck, tucking their chin back and pulling the head forward and down on their neck. As a result, the neck becomes too straight; the normal curvature flattens. This also compresses the vertebrae and disks. (See also Illustration II-2.)

4. Continue noticing what happens as you sit and stand by putting your hand on other areas of your body: lower back, abdomen, ribs, shoulders.

Do you find that you are using muscles you did not know you were using? For example, you do not need to tense your abdominal muscles as you sit or stand. You do not need to pull your shoulders up or down, grip your arms, squeeze your knees together, or hold your breath. You do not need to arch your back. Repeat this activity a number of times, discovering how you use your body as you move.

5. Another way to gather information about how you move is to do what Alexander did—watch yourself in a mirror.

If you have two standing mirrors, place them so that you can see your body in profile as you sit and stand. Observe your whole body as you move. Or ask a friend to film you as you sit and stand. What do you see?

6. Continue to notice how you move, especially how you move your head and neck as you do various activities: as you talk on the phone, lift a heavy object, brush your teeth, climb stairs, peel carrots, or ride a bicycle.

Once you are familiar with this process of self-observation, there is a lot to discover.

Can You Change?

1. **Put your hand on your head and neck again. Sit down and stand up, but this time try to do this *without* tensing your head and neck muscles in your usual way.**

   Were you able to *stop* tensing as you moved? Do not be alarmed if this was difficult. Not only do you not know a lot about your way of using your muscles, you have little control over this.

   Did you discover that in your effort to stop tensing you actually became tenser in other muscles? You are trying to prevent your muscles from tensing by tensing more!

   Did you notice emotional responses? Did you find yourself feeling annoyed, frustrated, or impatient? Did you feel worried or self-critical? These are common reactions to not being able to do what we try to do. It is normal to have these feelings and to be aware of them, but do not let your emotions discourage you from continuing on your new path of self-discovery.

2. **Place your hand on other parts of your body as you sit and stand. Try to stop tensing any unnecessary muscles. Notice what you do.**

   If you are like most people, you will find this surprisingly difficult.

▶ DISCUSSION

Most people know they are too tense. But in an effort to prevent this, they either tense more in other muscles, or relax all their muscles all at once. Neither excess muscle tension nor muscle relaxation is desirable when you move. *Moving with mastery means not using muscles that are not needed, while using the muscles that are—but only as much as necessary.* At every moment as you move, muscles should enter into and out of activity like the many musicians in an orchestra. This subtle, rapid adjustment and readjustment is highly complex. We all learn to move, but few of us learn to coordinate our muscles efficiently as we move.

Noticing Your Habit

1. Lie in semisupine with your left leg bent and your right leg straight on the floor. (See Illustration 12–1.)

2. Bend your right leg, bringing it next to your left leg and placing your foot on the floor. (Now you are in the semisupine position.) As you do this movement, notice which muscles work. Straighten your leg again and repeat the movement several times, collecting data about the muscles that you use as you bend your leg.

If you are not sure what you are doing, place your hands on the front of your pelvis to feel if it is rotating or tilting. Notice the feeling of your back on the floor, and whether your back shifts as you move your leg. Notice the contact of your other foot on the floor. Notice your shoulders. Does one shoulder press more downward, the other lift? Does your jaw tense? Does your neck tighten? What else do you notice?

3. Repeat the same movement with the other leg, noticing how you move.

Is there a difference between this leg and your other one?

Do you feel muscles working in your body other than in the leg that is moving? Since you are lying down, you only need to do a little work in the front of your hip and at the back of your knee to bend your leg. If you feel other muscles working, you are tensing muscles that you do not need.

4. Try to bend your leg without tensing the muscles that you do not need, as you did in the first experiment in this section when you tried to sit down and stand up without unnecessary muscular effort.

[Note: Throughout the remaining series of leg experiments, bend whichever leg you choose.]

It is likely that you find it difficult *not* to tense the muscles you do not need. You may have the thought that it is impossible to move your leg without tensing your back, abdomen, or neck muscles. You are discovering that you have a characteristic way of using your muscles as you bend your leg that you cannot change.

With these observations, you may wonder: Why do I move my leg with too much muscular effort? Is this solely a problem of my body? Is this my leg's fault? What makes this happen?

Your Mind-Body Connection

1. Lie in semisupine. Place one leg straight on the floor. Think to yourself, *I am not going to bend my leg*. Repeat this thought to yourself for several minutes.

    Did you feel the same muscle tension that you felt when you were moving your leg? (Of course not, because you did not move your leg!) Did you feel that your muscles continued to relax, more and more deeply, as you thought of not moving? If you did not feel this, try it again and give it plenty of time.

2. Put your leg straight on the floor. Decide to bend your leg and then bend it. Feel the familiar pattern of tension that is triggered. Do this several times.

    Notice that when you decide to move, you tense your muscles in your usual way.

3. Put your leg straight on the floor. Tell yourself to bend your leg, BUT DO NOT BEND IT. Have the thought in your mind—*decide* to bend your leg—but do not bend it. Notice what happens in your muscles.

    Can you feel your tension beginning as you decide to move? If you cannot feel this, decide to bend your leg and then move it a small amount. Notice the familiar pattern of tension that is triggered in your muscles as soon as you start to move. Try this several times. Can you notice that in the split second between when you decide to move, and the moment that you actually move, your tension begins?

    As this becomes easier to recognize, go back to deciding to move your leg without actually moving it. Can you feel that a split second after you have this thought, your muscles tense? In other words, your particular pattern of muscle tension begins *before* you move. Further, your muscle tension is triggered by your *thought* of moving.

▶ **DISCUSSION**

This simple experiment demonstrates two important things. First, if you tell yourself not to move, you do not trigger any muscle tension. In fact, if you continue thinking of not moving your leg for a while, you will feel your muscles letting go more and more. Second, when you decide to move, you tense your muscles in a specific and characteristic way. Your decision to move—your *thought* of doing the movement—is tied to the way that you use your muscles as you move. This simple experiment demonstrates the mind-body connection. Your thought to move creates a particular pattern of activity that is unique to you. You do not bend your leg the way your best friend does. In addition, there is a particular *way that you think*, which creates the particular *way that you move*. Thinking and moving are two parts of a whole, which is your behavior.

It is your thought that determines how you move, since if you do not think of moving, you do not tense. This means that you cannot change *how you move* until you change *how you think*. This is what you will explore in the next series of self-experiments.

HOW DO YOU FEEL?

THE MIND-BODY LINK

A Sense of Feeling

The mind's first step to self-awareness
must be through the body.
—GEORGE SHEEHAN

RECENTLY I WAS asked to teach a course on the Alexander Technique to undergraduate students at a nearby college. Today I have begun class by questioning the students about their senses.

"How many senses do you have?" I ask.

The group's unanimous tally is five: the well-known quintet of sight, sound, smell, taste, and touch.

"Do you know you have more than that?" I ask. The faces before me are blank. Not wanting to cause embarrassment, I hurry to explain.

"You have a sixth sense, but it is not ESP. I like to call it the sense of **bodily sensation**. We might also call it the sense of feeling. This comes to you from millions of **sensory receptors** spread throughout your body. These receptors send information to your brain to inform it of what is happening within you." As I talk, I watch for signs of interest in my students' faces.

"Your brain receives data from these many receptors that paint a broad palette of experience: the feeling that you're bending your knees and swinging your arms; that your muscles ache;

that your eyes are blinking, your skin itches, your stomach hurts, or you've got goose bumps. It includes much subtler sensations as well, such as the feeling that you know you are right or that you have forgotten something important.

"Your emotions also come to your awareness via this sixth sense of bodily sensation. How do you know you're sad or angry? You feel this, don't you? Isn't that why we speak of our emotions as feelings? Emotions are changes in brain states that produce neurological and biochemical changes that affect our body, especially our viscera. Due to this, sensory receptors are stimulated that send signals back to the brain with lightning speed, telling it about what is happening within us. Some of these signals reach conscious awareness. Then you say you feel your heart pounding and feel afraid, or that you feel queasy in your stomach and say you are nervous, or feel a grin spread across your face and say that you are ecstatic. But much of this bodily feedback is processed below the level of conscious awareness." Looking at my audience, I see they are intrigued.

"Synthesizing this vast array of bodily information, arriving at every moment, awake and asleep, your brain creates a construct of you. It adds up these inputs and generates a sense of the whole. More than any of your other senses, it is bodily sensation that enables your brain to construct a concept of **self**: Imagine a vastly complex matrix of neurons, neurotransmitters, and electrochemical signaling, changing instant to instant, yet creating a gestalt—your mind's concept of 'you.'

"This sixth sensory system of bodily sensation has been overlooked for the vital role it plays in our behavior. This is surprising when we consider that bodily sensations are at the root of most of what we know and believe about ourselves. Our self-concept is derived from this all-body rainbow of bodily feeling, much of which is triggered when we move and act.* In turn, this concept of *self* plays an essential role in shaping how we use our body to

---

* Both *kinesthesia* and *proprioception* are defined as our capacity to feel and be aware of our body in motion. (Proprioception is usually defined more broadly to include inputs from the vestibular apparatus.) Neither word is defined to include the feelings that come to us through our viscera—pounding heart, gurgling stomach, etc., that neuroscientists define as *interoception*; nor do these words encompass the sensations that we speak of as our emotions. Since there is no single word or phrase that defines the entire spectrum of bodily sensations of which we are capable, I have coined my own—the sense of *bodily sensation*—and labeled it our sixth sense. I use the words *feeling* and *bodily feedback* synonymously with this.

accomplish everything we do. For example, years ago you sat at your desk in school and were taught how to hold a pen and write. Gradually a sensory memory of writing was instilled in your brain and linked to your meaning of the word 'write.' Now all you have to do is pick up a pen and think of writing. Your mind activates your muscles in the way that feels like writing, just as it has been doing for decades. You don't think about how you write, you don't have to. You coordinate your muscles to grip your pen as you did when you were young because it *feels* like the right way to do it.

"Bodily sensation brings us an enormous array of information about ourselves, but we usually don't appreciate its importance because much of it is processed below the level of conscious awareness. The sensations we become aware of are the tip of the iceberg. Yet these inputs deeply affect our behavior. They're like music playing in the background. We can push it out of our awareness but it puts us in a certain mood.

"We also fail to realize that this sensory system limits what we think of as our free will. Once you have learned how to hold your pen and write, you can choose whether to write or not, but you can't choose to perform the act of writing differently. Have you ever tried to hold your pen in a new way? If you do, your mind will rebel. It will tell you that what you're doing doesn't feel right. It will invent any number of reasons to explain why you shouldn't or can't hold your pen in this new way. You'll soon find yourself reverting to your habitual way of writing, because it jibes with your brain's learned idea of how writing should feel.

"Another example is that, as I am standing here talking to you, I might be feeling sensations of anxiety. After all, I'm talking to a group of strangers, which can be scary. If these feelings are unpleasant enough, later I may decide that speaking to groups is something I don't like to do and decline the offer the next time I'm asked. Little may I realize that what I believe is a conscious choice amounts to a subconscious aversion to a memory of uncomfortable bodily feelings.

"The feelings that are generated within us as we do everything we do—from moving to thinking to remembering—not only shape how we move, they shape our **beliefs** about ourselves, and this in turn influences our actions and decisions.

"If you always sit in a slouch, eventually you will come to believe that this is 'how you sit.' If someone recommends that you sit more upright, you will say that this feels bad or feels wrong. Even though your slouch is injuring your spine, you will hold firmly to your belief that slouching is okay because it feels good to you. And you will probably hold to this belief no matter what you are told about the importance of sitting more upright.

"Perhaps at some point you've experienced a difficult, painful ending of a love affair. Months or even years later, a friend mentions this person's name and in an instant the thought of that individual now planted in your mind triggers a flood of biochemical changes in your body. Suddenly a mere thought is generating bodily feelings: you feel your heart pounding, your stomach churning, and a lump rising in your throat. You thought the relationship was over. It is, but the memory of this person still has the power to catapult you into a cascade of bodily experiences. In an effort to quell the discomfort plaguing you in the present moment you say to your friend, 'I don't want to talk about it.' But what you're really saying is, 'I don't like feeling this way. I want it to stop.' Later you may form the belief that talking about this old relationship is a bad idea, and flatly refuse when someone asks you to speak of it.

"To demonstrate the mysterious power of our sixth sense in determining how we perceive ourselves and form beliefs about ourselves, would someone like to volunteer to lie down on this table?" Liz, a perky young woman with curly hair and a ready smile shoots up her hand.

"Liz? You want to try this? Great. Lie down on your back. Everyone else can gather around to watch as we conduct a bit of an experiment. Liz, bend your left knee and put your left foot on the table. Then put your right leg down straight. I'm going to slightly lift your right leg and support it for you. While I do this, think to yourself of not holding on to your leg. Allow me to support it."

The class is silent, watching.

"I'm lifting and very slightly moving your leg, but you don't have to do anything. Just think of not holding on to your leg." Liz nods. A few moments later, I put her leg down. A smile spreads across her face.

"Yes?" I ask, inviting comment.

"This isn't my leg!" Liz blurts out, giggling. "This is so strange! What happened? This isn't my leg," she repeats.

Looking at the students standing around the table I ask, "What does she mean when she says, 'This isn't my leg'? Did I take off the old one and replace it with a new one?" Everyone laughs.

"Of course not. Then why does she say this? Her choice of words seems surprising; but if we think about it, they tell us a lot about how her mind has processed the **sensory feedback** she just experienced. First, she's experiencing a new sensation. Is that a fair statement, Liz?"

"Yes!"

"Isn't this interesting. She didn't say, 'This feeling is different from anything I've felt before.' She said, 'This isn't my leg!' Why does she express it this way? Years ago her mind formed an idea of what a leg is—based on how she felt as she moved her leg and generated sensations in her muscles and joints. Now it's as if there's a file folder on the desktop in her mind that's labeled, 'my right leg.' Contrasting this with the new feeling that I generated when I supported her leg, her mind shuffled through the leg folder but nothing linked up. The remembered feeling of leg didn't jibe with this new feeling. Her choice of words is very apt, because in a sense to her mind this is exactly right. It's not the felt sense of her leg, as she knows it. So her mind took a guess to explain it: 'Maybe it's someone else's!'

"Anyone else want to try?" Hands shoot up. "Dan, let's have you get on the table." Liz gets off while Dan walks to the front of the room. Dan has been a quiet member of the group, and I am unsure how he is responding to the material. I am surprised that he has volunteered and curious to see how he reacts. I ask him to lie down, bend both knees, and place his hands on his ribs. Next I put my left hand under his right elbow to lift his arm slightly, and then I take hold of his right hand in my right hand. Slowly I straighten Dan's elbow, extending his arm. Repeating a similar process of lifting and supporting, I ask Dan to think of not holding on to his arm. I remain in this position for a few minutes. Then, as I feel a subtle sensation of release in his musculature, I guide his arm slightly away from his body. I repeat this process a few times without talking.

Although I have not asked him to volunteer any comments, Dan suddenly speaks. "This is amazing!"

"What's amazing?"

"My arm feels like it's a couple of inches longer! How'd you do that?"

Without changing my position, I turn to the group and ask, "Does it look like his arm is a couple of inches longer?"

"No!" They answer in unison, smiling.

I look at Dan. His expression is serious. "This feels kind of scary," he says quietly.

I put his arm down in its original position. "Does anything hurt?"

"No, not at all. It feels good."

"Why do you say it feels scary?"

"I don't know. It's so different from the way my arm usually feels. It feels light and loose. It's different from what I'm used to, I guess."

"You see?" I say, looking at the group. "Like Liz, Dan's mind doesn't know what to make of these new feelings. His mind has also filled in the blank, but differently. First, he wondered if his arm had gotten longer. Rationally we know this isn't possible, but this is his mind's best guess to explain the new feeling. Then it added an emotion to the feeling—scary. This is common. The mind often interprets new bodily feelings by giving them emotional meaning.

"These are good examples of what I'm talking about. Your mind is interpreting sensory data all the time. If these feelings are *familiar*, your mind doesn't take much notice. But if they are *unfamiliar*, they get your mind's attention and it tries to figure out what they mean. But to say that a leg isn't your own, or that a new feeling is scary, is more than just an observation that a feeling is different. These are judgments, beliefs. We make decisions and base our behavior on them. If we decide that something is scary—even just a simple movement—we might avoid doing it again. Bodily sensations, and the judgments that flow from them, are a powerful team that drive our decisions and behavior, but we're largely unaware of this happening within us.

"Perhaps now we can better appreciate that our sixth sense is also linked to how we reason. Imagine someone saying to you, 'Let's go to the local swimming hole and jump off that twenty-foot cliff into the water. I was watching some kids doing it the other day. It looks like fun. Come on and try it with me.' As you silently consider your response, how do you feel? Do you feel excited by the thought of jumping twenty feet into the water? Or do you feel uneasy as you consider the possibility that you might slip and fall, and seriously injure yourself? In an instant your mind is summoning memories of previous experiences that evoke subtle sensations—pleasant or unpleasant feelings—tied to your mind's projection of what this experience will be. As a result, your decision will be influenced more than you realize not by cold, objective reasoning, but by bodily feelings arising within you in the present moment. Reasoning is in fact an experiential, personal, and physical process.[1]

"What is perhaps more surprising—when you consider how central this sensory system is to our beliefs and behavior—is that we are entirely unschooled in interpreting the meaning of our bodily sensations, or developing a greater awareness of the judgments and beliefs we form from them. The artist spends years training the acuity of her powers of observation. The musician learns to hear the subtlest variations in pitch, resonance, and expressiveness of sound. The chef tastes a food many times, deepening his skill at perceiving its shadings of flavor and learning to perceive the subtle nuances it produces in combination with other foods.

"Has anyone taught you to pay attention to this sensory language within yourself and to understand its message? To acquire skill in knowing the meaning of the feelings that are triggered within you as you move and as you live as a means for better understanding yourself? Or to appreciate the difficulty of changing your beliefs, precisely because they are tied to the feelings you experience as you move your body in your habitual way?"

My students remain silent as they watch me struggling to find a special eloquence that will sum this up for them. I seek a light in their eyes letting me know that, through these few demonstrations, a glimmer of understanding has penetrated. Of course, I realize this is only a beginning. Students must discover the role of bodily sensation in shaping their beliefs and behavior for themselves, gradually, over the course of many lessons. Mere words cannot fill the gap caused by faulty self-perception and the absence of conscious education. Still, I try to shine a light of understanding for them—and perhaps for myself as well—into the complicated interplay between how we move, how we feel, and what we believe.

6

Feelings Gone Wrong

Everyone wants to be right,
but no one stops to consider if
their idea of right is right.
—F. M. ALEXANDER

GARY

GARY CAME TO me for lessons to improve his piano playing.
He had a tendency, he said, to sound "rather bangy." To get some
idea of what he meant by this, I asked him to play for me. Soon
I understood his point: "bangy" was just the word that came to
mind to describe his unpleasing sound, despite his obvious facility at the keyboard. As I watched, I noticed numerous difficulties in his psychophysical coordination writ large upon his body.
Until he made headway in changing this, I knew he would not
achieve his goal.

I told him we were going to shift gears for the time being, and
I asked him to stand facing the mirror in my teaching room. As
he stood before me, I saw that his shoulders were uneven—the
left one oddly lifted and pulled into his neck. Neither of his arms
hung at his sides in anything resembling a straight line. His left
arm was distinctly flexed at the elbow and wrist, and the fingers
of both hands had a pronounced curl. I stood next to him facing the mirror. I asked if he saw any difference between his arms

and mine. We were both silent as his eyes moved from my image to his own. After a few moments he replied, "Not really."

I was so surprised by his answer that I stammered for a moment, not knowing what to say. Because of his extreme arm and shoulder tension, I did not expect that he would be able to feel this tension as he played. I did think, however, that he would be able to see the distortion in the alignment of his arms in the mirror, especially when faced with a ready source of comparison. But for Gary, seeing was not believing.

Over the course of more than a year of weekly lessons, I gently presented Gary with incontrovertible data. I showed him anatomy books, explained the structure of the arm and its movements, and showed him the arms on my life-sized model skeleton. I let him feel my arms as they moved. I gave him stretches to do at home. I worked with him sitting and standing, lying down, walking, and playing the piano. At the start of each lesson I asked him what he had noticed during the previous week. Each time he shrugged and told that me he had not noticed anything. Every week his arms and his entire body were as tight as the week before. My every tactic seemed to fall off him unheard, unseen, unfelt, as though he were vacuum-sealed.

I was baffled. Gary simply did not register the inner world of sensation. He did not feel his tension or feel how his arms moved, and so nothing I said meant anything to him. I considered telling him I could not teach him, but decided instead to trust that, since he came for his lessons regularly, something must be penetrating.

One day Gary arrived with a smile on his face as he announced, "I've had a bit of an insight since our last lesson."

"What's that?" I asked.

"You want me to think about what I'm doing while I'm doing it," he said with a tone of pride.

Once again, my student left me speechless. This is such a basic concept of the Technique that most students grasp it in their first lesson. Gary had been coming for a long time and he was by no means unintelligent. I did my best to hide my true reaction, and expressed instead my pleasure at his discovery.

After that lesson, however, Gary began reporting regularly on his observations and discoveries. It seemed he had finally stumbled onto his sixth sense, like finding an old pair of shoes in the back of the closet.

A few months later Gary arrived for his lesson with a particularly bright face, letting me know there was something he wanted to say.

"Yes?" I asked.

"An amazing thing happened this week. I was standing at my worktable a few nights ago. I happened to look down, and I saw that my left arm was pulled in against my side and bent just as you've been telling me."

Unsure of my best response, I asked him what he did next.

"My wife was in the room with me and I asked her to look at my arm."

"What did she say?"

"She told me I always hold my arm like that! So I asked her, 'Why haven't you told me this before?'"

"What did she say?"

"She told me she didn't want to hurt my feelings!"

I was silent for a moment, filled with the poignancy of his story. "You have a kind wife," I said.

For weeks afterward, Gary's story kept coming back to me, his wife's words replaying themselves in my mind. She had understood. She knew her husband well. As I had discovered all too slowly, it had not done any good to tell him about his arms. He literally could not comprehend this information. Gary's chronic tension had not just skewed his awareness of bodily feelings; it had shut it down. Yet somehow the lessons had had an accumulating effect. Like a bear slowly waking from hibernation, Gary began to hear the nonverbal language playing within him.

From that lesson, Gary became an eager and apt student. He changed. He practiced. He made his own connections and enjoyed his emerging self-awareness. Had I stopped teaching him, I would have denied both of us the pleasure of his discovery of the mysterious and sometimes hard-to-find realm of the self.

~

GARY IS AN extreme example. Few people are so unable to listen to the physical realm. Such people are uncommon and they usually do not choose to come for Alexander lessons, or continue for long when they do. For those who do take lessons, awakening their awareness of bodily sensation is the first task. Such individuals have devised complex strategies for keeping feelings at bay. The lessons gradually help to remove this interference, but if they are pushed before they are ready they will resist. If a student cannot feel something he is doing that is causing a particular problem, he literally cannot comprehend what the teacher is saying. He can hear and know the dictionary meaning of individual words, but he has not yet forged a *connection* between these words, the felt experience of his body, and his concept of himself. As Gary's story shows, it is especially difficult for some individuals to grasp the importance of bodily sensation—a sensory system they seem never to have known.

For most us, however, our sixth sense presents a different problem. Unlike the information that comes to us from our other senses, the data we receive from our sixth sense is not so indelibly cast: Once learned, the color red is red. The sound of C sharp is C sharp. The taste of salt is salty. But bodily feelings can shift and change.

The next story shows the havoc that our feelings, which often lie hidden within us and whisper falsehoods in our brains, can create.

BETTY, PART ONE

Betty is a short, slightly rounded woman of middle age. She has come to me complaining of pain in her hips when she walks for any length of time. Today, a few months into her lessons, I have asked her to stand facing the mirror in my teaching room.

"Betty, I'd like you to watch yourself as you shift your weight onto your right leg, and then take a step forward on your left." Observing her in the mirror, I see that Betty begins to move by pushing her pelvis too far to the right. Then, in order to counterbalance herself, she pulls her upper body to the left. This causes her right leg—the leg she wants to stand on—to tilt to the right so that it is no longer perpendicular to the ground but leaning at an angle. Now that she has pulled her body out of balance, she lifts her left leg with visible effort and takes a step (see Illustration 6-1).

"Betty, was there anything that you noticed as you observed yourself moving?" Betty's face is blank. She is searching for something to say, but it is clear she does not understand the point of my question.

"I just did as you asked," she replies.

"Nothing unusual caught your eye?"

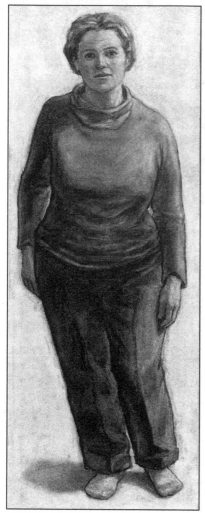

6-1. Betty standing on her right leg and taking a step with the left leg. Her pelvis is collapsing to the right and her upper torso is leaning to the left, tilting her torso. Her right leg is leaning sideward, her right shoulder is lifted, and her right arm is pulled back; her head is also tilted. The left knee is pulled inward.

"No."

"Okay, good," I offer in encouragement as I consider what to say next. Rather than explain to Betty that she is pulling herself seriously off balance, creating a significant sheering, compression force on her right hip and overtensing her back muscles, I decide to continue our exploration.

"Betty, let's do this again. This time I'm going to help you."

I stand behind her with my hands on her lower ribs. I ask her to allow me to move her torso slightly, shifting her body over her right leg. I explain that, as I am doing this she does not have to do anything, only to think of not helping me. I repeat my instructions, emphasizing that the shift onto her right leg is only a few inches. She nods in acknowledgment.

With a light touch I guide Betty's torso until she is standing over her right foot. I continue supporting her gently with my hands. Her right leg is upright, perpendicular to the ground. Her torso is vertical and her head is directly over her foot. I ask her again to bend her left leg and take a step, but Betty does not move. Her eyes shift downward as if she is trying to see inside herself. Her face tells me the story of her thoughts—Betty thinks I have asked the impossible.

"Go ahead," I urge her gently, "I'm supporting you so you can't fall. Bend your left leg and take a step."

Betty looks bewildered. Her eyes are still downward. Her attention is focused on the new feelings she is experiencing. These are different, and she does not know what they mean. "I can't take a step," she says after a moment, "I'm not standing on my leg."

Betty's choice of words reveals how her mind has processed these new feelings. She does not feel as she usually does when she stands on her leg, and so her mind has wrongly concluded that she must not be standing on her leg.

"Look in the mirror, Betty. Your head and torso are directly over your right leg and your foot is on the ground, right?"

"I guess so," she says hesitantly.

"You are standing on your leg, you're just standing on it differently. Go ahead and take a step. I'm supporting you so you can't fall. Give it a try."

In the next instant everything changes. Betty's jaw muscles tense. She pushes her pelvis to the right, pulls her upper body to the left, and takes a step. She has made her body do exactly what it did before.

"Betty, what happened? Why did you pull yourself over like that? I said I'd support you. You saw in the mirror that you were standing, balanced on your leg."

"I had to shift my weight like that so I could take a step," she answers.

How can this be? How can a normal, intelligent woman hold steadfastly to her belief despite what I have explained and what she has seen in the mirror? Why is she convinced that the only way to stand on her leg is to push her body off balance, tense muscles she does not need, further compressing already painful joints, and making the task more difficult than it needs to be?

When I press her for an explanation she repeats herself. "I feel as though I can't move my left leg or I'll fall," she says, letting me know by her tone that she is right.

But Betty is not right. She is misinterpreting the meaning of her feelings. Despite seeing herself in the mirror, my hands supporting her, and my explanations, Betty does not believe what she has seen or heard. She only believes her mind's sensory judgment.

Betty is not suffering from dementia. She is not delusional. She does not have some odd neurological disorder. But her words give us an important glimpse into how her mind has interpreted these feelings and the judgment it has formed. Contrasted against the feelings she usually has when she stands on one leg, this new way of standing and my argument for it hold no weight. Her view of the matter is all that she can comprehend. It does not occur to her to question her judgment. In the grip of her belief, she cannot move or think differently than she has always done. Her mind is absorbed by the sensations from her body and her belief about their meaning. It is her *belief* that determines how she stands, far more than her *muscles* do. This misjudgment may seem minor but it governs her every step.

BETTY'S COMPLAINT OF pain when she walks and Gary's complaint of sounding bangy when he plays are not simply physical problems. Gary cannot improve his playing by practicing more. Betty's hip problem cannot be cured by walking less, or by exercising more. These are psychophysical problems, caused by how the mind interprets bodily sensation, and its all-too-frequent tendency to interpret this data incorrectly.

These sensory errors fall into four categories: 1) *Filling in the blank.* As we have seen in the example of my students in the theater class, new sensations are an unfamiliar experience and the mind takes a guess to explain them. Liz thought the new feeling meant that it was not her leg. Dan thought it meant that his arm was longer. 2) *Adding emotional content.* In Dan's case, his sensory misjudgment included an emotional tag. He labeled the new feeling scary. 3) *Blocking.* By contrast, Gary's mind learned not to pay attention to bodily sensation. Feelings that others could readily experience, he did not consciously register. 4) *Misjudging.* Betty's story shows that what seems to feel right may actually be wrong, and vice versa. She thought she was balanced on her leg when she was seriously out of balance. These misjudgments keep her locked in her harmful way of moving, compounding her pain and injury.

In summary, our mind learns from bodily sensations. Then it forms beliefs about their meaning, usually below the level of our conscious awareness, and these beliefs shape our behavior. Once the brain has formed such beliefs, changing how we behave is more difficult than we realize. To do this, we must change the beliefs that drive the behavior, and so, too, the sensations (feelings) from which these beliefs arise. And what is the prime source of our bodily sensations? *It is how we move and use our bodies.* Before we go on to learn how the Technique teaches us to use our locomotor system more skillfully and so to change how we feel and thus how we perceive ourselves, there is more to understand about our feelings— particularly our feelings of fear.

7

The Feeling of Fear

No passion so effectually robs the mind of all its powers
of acting and reasoning as fear.
—EDMUND BURKE

WALKING DOWN THE wooded path we have traveled a
hundred times before, I marvel at my companion, Burleigh,
a large male standard poodle. He trots briskly as I note his supple spine, the action of his legs, and the strong, wide paws pushing powerfully against the earth to propel him forward. Burleigh
has an unflagging interest in everything around him. Occasionally his tail signals a dash of joy as he doubles back to follow a
scent, pauses, and rushes off again, following an invisible trail.
Now he stops and looks for me, finding me on the path ahead.
I give a short whistle and Burleigh bounds back, hopping over
small shrubs and logs, more kangaroo than canine.

This is all part of our routine, but today something not so routine happens. Some distance ahead I see another dog and his
owner walking toward us. My dog is large. The other dog is massive. I reach out to grab Burleigh by the collar to restrain him
before he notices the other animal, but I am too late. In the second before I close my grasp, he has caught the scent. Burleigh
dashes ahead as the other dog moves briskly forward to meet

him, unrestrained. I follow behind hoping these dogs—strangers to one another—will negotiate an amicable greeting.

When they are about twenty feet apart, Burleigh stops and stands, frozen. The other dog slows to a walk. As he nears, Burleigh's neck and tail droop. In order to continue watching the other dog, however, he pulls his head back to raise his eyes. The other dog moves forward slowly, cautiously. He too lowers his neck and pulls his head back. Burleigh drops his neck farther as he bends his forelegs, lowering his upper body. He looks like a supplicant. The other dog approaches within four feet and stops. He growls—a rumbling, ominous sound. Neither dog moves. I am unmoving myself, not knowing whether to intervene or how.

Suddenly the other dog shows his teeth and bursts into loud, fast barks. He lunges forward, jaws snapping. Burleigh responds in an instant by spinning around and running, tail pulled tightly between his legs. His run is awkward, impeded by the tension of his fear. When he reaches me he stops on a dime, kicking up a rain of dirt, and turns to face the other dog. Burleigh lies down at my feet, flattening his body into the ground. In the time it has taken him to do this the other dog has reached us. Burleigh rolls over, belly up. The other dog stops one foot away and lowers his head, reaching forward for a leisurely sniff. Burleigh is still lying on his back in submission as they touch tentatively—one nose right side up, the other upside down.

The other dog's owner catches up but continues walking. He calls his dog as he smiles at me noncommittally. He is not apologizing, and he is not pretending his dog has not had the upper hand. Soon they are behind us. Burleigh rolls over and sits. I bend down to give him a reassuring pat. He leans heavily against my leg. We resume our walk, but Burleigh does not bounce off into the bushes. He trots slowly, staying near me, head lowered, tail down. His enthusiasm for discovery has dimmed.

ONE MORNING A few years ago I was feeling especially calm and relaxed. The kids were in school. Burleigh, at that time an adorable four-month-old puppy, was sleeping in the kitchen. It was a bright, spring day. Since I had a break in my teaching schedule I decided to relish the moment with a book. I lay down on the sofa, propped my head, and began to read. Perhaps because I was so relaxed, what happened next seemed to unfold as a series of separate events, as if a moment in time had been split into separate scenes for slow motion, frame-by-frame viewing. In less than a second this is what happened.

Out of the corner of my eye, my brain identified something unusual on the carpet: something brown and lumpy. My neck muscles contracted forcefully, yanking my head to the left. As my head turned there was a surging queasiness in my gut and my heart began pounding hard. My arms felt prickly as the hairs stood up. Not knowing what was wrong, or why I was behaving this way, my eyes turned to align the fearsome object in the center of my field of vision for identification. The threat was located and brought into focus—a brown leather shoe.

Now conscious awareness caught up with events, merging them into a cohesive whole. My unconscious mind had guessed that the brown, lumpy object was an accident left by our puppy, threatening to damage the new carpet. I had had a powerful fear reaction, but my fear was misplaced. The silliness of my behavior struck home. I burst into laughter as sensations of relief welled up . . . no cleanup necessary, no damage done.

Returning to my book, I found I could not concentrate. Although I understood my error, the remnants of this powerful reaction still filled me, disturbing my body and mind: pounding heart; queasy stomach; and quivering muscles. No wonder I could not think—my mind was preoccupied by all this bodily sensation. I decided to conduct an experiment—to stay on the sofa observing myself until this raucous band of feelings ceased its cacophony. To my amazement, it was over half an hour before their last notes ceased to play.

HOW WE PERCEIVE DANGER

Amygdala. Have you ever heard of it? It is not a tiny country on a faraway continent, an exotic tuberous root with mysterious powers, or a rare disease. But we can characterize it as a small, unknown territory, a conjuror of inexplicable behavior, and the source of many of our ills. The amygdala resides within us. To be precise, it is tucked away in our forebrain, symmetrically paired and almond shaped, deep in the medial area of the temporal lobes. The amygdala is our sentry that never sleeps. It follows us wherever we go, watching every circumstance for danger. Its purpose is to evaluate incoming **sensory stimuli** for threats to the organism. Then it triggers a series of physical and mental changes that propel us like a train on its track into behaviors of defense. Let us see the part my amygdala played in this story of mistaken identity.

As I was reading, my amygdala was standing ready. A visual stimulus arrived at my visual cortex and was routed onward to my amygdala: "Hello! There's something unusual on the floor. What do you think?"

In a flash the amygdala rendered its appraisal: "Looks dangerous! Sound the alarm!"

Neurological messages were sent careering outward via the nerves of the **sympathetic nervous system** to my viscera as well as via **motor nerves** to the muscles of my locomotor system. In an instant, a full-organism, **neurochemical response** was triggered. My heart beat faster and harder. Blood vessels dilated to allow increased blood flow to the muscles, readying them for action. Digestion slowed. The adrenal glands increased adrenalin production for muscle strength and mental alertness. Respiration increased. Blood pressure rose, and much more. This is often referred to as our **fight-or-flight response**, which has long been observed by scientists, but thanks largely to the groundbreaking research of Joseph LeDoux, a neuroscientist at New York University, the role of the amygdala and the brain's neural pathways of defense have been traced.[1]

This rapid, neurochemical signaling is not the end of the story. It is just the first act, setting the stage for a larger purpose: launching us into self-defense behavior. Vertebrates have four **stereotyped defense behaviors**, which we witnessed in Burleigh's story: 1) *Attack,* or threaten the enemy. 2) *Freeze,* tensing muscles to stop movement and avoid the enemy's notice. 3) *Withdraw,* moving away from the enemy. 4) *Submit,* yielding to the enemy like the docile subject of a tyrannical ruler.[2]

In each of these behaviors, the locomotor system is an essential vehicle of our defense. In my own case, first my head and eyes were oriented to the object as my mind went into hyperalert and every muscle became taut. Then I froze. If my brain had supposed the object to be a snake, I would have leaped up from the sofa like a popped cork and run for the door. Burleigh's first reaction was to freeze, but after the other dog growled and snapped at him, he withdrew. Then he rolled over and exposed his belly, submitting to his aggressor.

Once a defense behavior has been activated, sensory receptors throughout our body are stimulated. Bodily sensations begin flooding back to the brain, informing the brain of our defensive action: *I'm running.*

This bodily feedback may also be routed on to the amygdala, which may interpret it as meaning a further threat. In turn, the amygdala may generate further defensive behavior: *Keep running.*

The amygdala may also decide that a particular stimulus means the threat is even more dangerous than previously thought, and send commands to boost our energy level: *Run faster.*

As we saw in the previous chapter, because of bodily sensations our conscious mind can become aware of what we are doing. However, this happens *after* we have been triggered into a defense behavior. My body went into its freeze reaction because my subconscious mind saw the object and my amygdala appraised it as a threat, not because I was consciously aware of feeling afraid and decided what to do. Like a passenger on a bus who feels its sudden, veering motion only after the driver has pulled sharply on the wheel, "I" was the last to know what was happening.

This seems counterintuitive but it is vital. Awareness and decision making have an important role, but in the face of immediate, life-threatening danger split seconds can mean all the difference. The luxury of self-awareness is kept in abeyance while action is summoned. In short, I did not choose and could not control this neurochemical activity and stereotyped locomotor behavior in myself. Nor could I decide to turn off its lingering sensory aftermath.

As immediate danger abates, what happens next—especially in humans—might be described as a second tier of defense. Feelings rise to our awareness, and higher cortical areas of the brain come into play. Paired with our capacity for using language to describe and reflect on our behavior and circumstances, we have further options.

We can name our emotions/feelings: "My heart is pounding. I'm feeling scared."

As we have seen, the sensations we call *fear* are the result of our mind's interpretation of bodily feedback. These sensations are different from those of joy or confusion, for example. We learn to name the feelings that we call our emotions. It is not the function of the amygdala to give us the ability to feel fear specifically or to feel emotion in general. It is to detect threats and generate defensive behavior. We can only know that we are afraid or threatened to the extent that we become aware of, and then correctly identify the bodily stamp of amygdala activity.

If this feedback is weak, more subtly varied, slower to arise, or if it comes at the same time that we are feeling other competing sensations or our attention is distracted, we may describe ourselves as feeling anxious, uneasy, stressed out, tense, or on edge. Or we may feel nothing. A wide range of feelings can indicate that something has triggered our amygdala into action. But these bodily sensations mean that, whether or not we describe ourselves as afraid, our amygdala has propelled us into some degree and type of defense behavior.

Although we may not recognize our feelings as meaning we are in a state of fear, due to conscious awareness we can notice our behavior. Our mind seeks the reason for our actions. By drawing on judgment, experience, and knowledge, we seek to explain our actions to ourselves and to others. *We create a self-story to explain our behavior:* "Yesterday the dog had four accidents in the house. Wouldn't YOU be paranoid?"

We may also override our first defense behavior and make another, more conscious choice: "I don't need to do anything. It was a false alarm. I'll just stay on the sofa and relax."

These examples give us a glimpse into our **self-defense system**, which is two-tiered. Operating below conscious awareness, the first tier of defense consists of a sensory stimulus, the amygdala's appraisal of the stimulus, a neurochemical response, a stereotyped defense behavior played out via our viscera and our locomotor system, and bodily sensation or feedback. In the second tier, consciousness of our feelings brings awareness of something that has changed within us and in our behavior. Combined with language and self-reflection, this gives us further options. We can recognize bodily sensations, name our feelings, create a self-story to explain our behavior, and make a different conscious choice.

Thus far I have painted a picture of a defense system that is functioning well. Next we will look at how this system goes awry due to long-term activation of the amygdala, causing what is commonly known as **anxiety**. We will see how this anxiety wreaks havoc on our locomotor system, and on our physical and mental health.

8

Fear's Body-Mind

To him who is in fear everything rustles.
—SOPHOCLES

IN THE GRIP OF FEAR

TODAY I HAVE a new student. On the telephone a week
before, she explained to me that her physician gave her an alarming diagnosis—severe osteoporosis. In addition to recommending medication, he suggested she study the Alexander Technique,
explaining that although it would not cure her condition, it could
teach her to maintain a more balanced, upright poise of her head,
neck, and spine to reduce pressure on her vertebrae and perhaps
prevent stress fractures.

As Joan sits facing me she adds, "My doctor told me I have terrible posture. I know I do. I know it will help if I can do something about that."

I smile and nod my head. Then I ask if she has any other complaints or problems.

"Well," she says hesitantly, hunching her shoulders and pulling
her head back as if ducking beneath a low doorframe, "a while
ago there was a crisis in my life. It stressed me out. Afterward I

began to have panic attacks." Still in her ducking pose, Joan tucks her hands under her thighs.

"They have been somewhat better in the last six months, but now they're happening again. This diagnosis hasn't helped. I'm worried about fractures. I've tried therapy, acupuncture, antidepressants, yoga. Nothing seems to help. My yoga teacher tells me to focus on my breathing, which I try to do. But some days I wake up and feel like I can't breathe. Then I know I'm going to have a bad day. I try to focus on remembering to breathe. Maybe it helps a little, but I don't want to have to keep reminding myself to breathe."

Joan, an older Asian woman with medium-length black hair streaked gray, smiles, but it is not an expression of happiness. I feel saddened by her story and wonder what lies behind it. As I nod my head in sympathy, she pulls her knees tightly together and presses her lips into a thin line. While we have been talking her muscles have been called into contraction, the contraction of freeze. Her bright eyes flit upward to glance at me and then drop downward. I have a brief glimpse of struggle, determination, and courage.

What has happened to give her reason to learn this?

Joan is not saying it out loud, but observing her body I see that this bright, vibrant woman is struggling to swim against a swelling tide of fear. I realize that my every word and action holds the potential to be a stimulus for more.

I help Joan to sit on my teaching table and lie down. I ask if she is comfortable, and to let me know if anything makes her feel uneasy. Proceeding slowly, I am conscious that everything I say and do must first be aimed at giving her a sense of safety and creating trust in order not to compound her state of fear. For now, all else is secondary.

I place my hands on the sides of her head and neck. The muscles in her neck protrude like ropes. I notice a shortening on the right side of her neck and an asymmetry in her face. Her extreme tension is misaligning her jaw. I apply the slightest pressure to turn her head, and ask her to think of not tightening her neck muscles to let me do this, but her head doesn't move. I lift her head slightly. It feels heavy in my hands—another sign of her excessive tension.

Proceeding to Joan's shoulders, arms, and legs, I repeat a similar procedure as I ask her to think of not holding on to her body. As I speak, my hands seek to feel her response. They bring me vital information that cannot be seen. Joan's body feels as if it has been compressed into a tiny space. She barely breathes. I watch her face for clues, seeking to know if she understands what I am asking, and whether I am provoking further anxiety. Gradually her muscles soften under my hands. Her limbs become lighter and her expression eases.

"Any problems?" I ask.

"No, I feel okay," she says with a slight smile.

After a half hour I help her to sit up on the table. Before I can help her to standing, she begins talking.

"About six months ago I tried some massage."

Why didn't she mention this before?

"After the first session I felt relaxed. Sort of like the way I feel now," she adds. "Then after the second session, I had a panic attack. The session after that, I had an even bigger one. So I decided I'd better stop."

Why does something that makes her feel good trigger a panic attack?

Not wanting to challenge her, I let her comments pass and continue with the lesson. Later as we finish, I see that Joan is wearing a real smile. "I feel good," she says with a tone of surprise.

I suggest that she spend the rest of the day taking it easy rather than doing errands. "This is a slow process of learning to change. Don't expect too much of it—or yourself—too quickly. The good feeling you're having now will fade. Don't try to hold on to it."

Joan smiles but instead of responding to my comment, she launches into a topic of her own. "I've tried a lot of psychotherapy for this you know."

Since she's feeling better, Joan wants to talk. I sit down next to her instead of urging her out the door, silently inviting her to continue. "They ask you to trust them, and open up to them, but they just sort of sit there and stare at you. I don't feel comfortable at all." She pauses. "This isn't like that," she says with a shy smile.

"They always want me to tell them about the troubles I've had," she continues. "They expect me to open up to them immediately. That's the last thing they make me want to do. I know what I've been through. I'm not an idiot. I've seen everything in my life. Everything." Joan pauses as I watch the new ease and relaxation in her body vanish, replaced suddenly by a grim expression as her neck juts forward. As if commenting on the weather she adds, "As a girl

I was physically abused." Joan's eyes drop as her mouth tenses again. I wait, unspeaking.

"But I can't tell them these things!" she says with energy, looking me in the eye again. She pauses. Then she strains to take a breath and I notice the cords springing up in her neck. Speaking softly as if to herself she adds, "Why is it I am telling you?"

A THREATENING INJURY

Jim is in his mid-thirties. He has a slender build, short brown hair that is receding from his brow, and a neat, tidy appearance. He is a singer with a problem. Two years ago he suffered damage to his vocal cords and was advised to stop singing. Sitting in my teaching room, Jim tells me that the throat specialist said he is recovered. Nevertheless, he is having difficulty getting back into his singing. He is sure, he says, knitting his eyebrows and leaning forward as if to imprint his difficulty on my mind, that something is still not right with his voice.

"But the specialist looked at your throat and told you everything is healed?" I ask, reframing his words.

"Yes."

Why doesn't he believe his physician?

Knowing that telling Jim to trust his doctor will not address his problem, I begin from another angle. "Would you sing a note for me? Any note."

A vibrant sound fills the room, which in the first split second I hear it makes me think, *This is doing all right.* In the next fraction of a second the sound shifts. It is not bad, but it is definitely less spacious, less resonant.

"Okay, now stop."

Jim closes his mouth and turns to look at me. "You see?" is written in his eyes.

Instead of meeting his silent challenge I ask, "Can you say what you were thinking as you sang the note?"

"Well," he says after a moment, "shortly after I began I started listening to my sound. As I did that I felt something tighten in my throat and I began thinking about that. I thought it might be a tension that could reinjure my voice."

"Would you say you were worrying?" I ask.

Jim's eyes look away and his jaw tenses. "Yeah."

Stimulus and Appraisal

The first event that launches our defense system into action is a stimulus. Typically, we think of danger coming from our environment: a bus passing too close as we cross the street; a stranger behind us as we walk alone late at night; a sudden, loud noise; a burning smell. But threats can also arise from feelings within our body. Physical pain is the most obvious example, but a wide array of bodily sensations may be assessed by the amygdala as threatening: a feeling of a lump in your throat, an odd feeling in your stomach, a feeling of dizziness, even a new feeling that you have never had before.

Another type of internal threat arises from our own thoughts: the memory of a project at work that you did not handle well; the thought of an argument you had recently with a friend; a nagging sense that you left the oven on.

The mind cannot will us to be afraid, but it can summon a painful memory, a fleeting worried thought, a nervous anticipation, a voice of self-criticism. In a flash we have engaged our amygdala, which sends out its all-body signal of alarm. Although they seem innocent enough, such thoughts are stimuli that trigger our body into a defense response. In addition, we often play these thoughts over and over in our mind, as if expecting an answer.

Each worried thought Joan related to me in recounting her history acted as another threatening self-stimulus, becoming another deposit·into her personal bank of fear. The thought of her diagnosis was a threat, as were the pleasing (although unfamiliar) sensations of relaxation produced by the massage sessions, and especially her memories of long-ago events. As I worked with her, I saw and felt the effects of these fear-thoughts drawn starkly across the canvas of her body. Joan's every muscle was locked in *freeze*, pulling her ever inward upon herself. This state of chronic fear had exacted a heavy toll: tension so extreme she could barely breathe or move, chronic anxiety beyond the reach of physicians or therapists. *A limitless array of thoughts and bodily sensations can act as stimuli that are routed to the amygdala and appraised as threats—even sensations that do not reach the level of consciousness, and thoughts of which we are barely aware.*

Acting as judge and jury, the amygdala appraises stimuli and assigns them meaning: dangerous, not dangerous, or somewhere in between. But these are not objective and rational assessments. If I have had a good night's sleep, my life is in order and I feel well, a sudden banging noise in the house is greeted with curiosity as I wonder what my son is doing. If I am worried how I will make the next month's mortgage payment, have backache, and feel distracted by other problems, the same noise may produce a gasp of startled reaction as my shoulders hunch and my first angry thought is, "What is he doing NOW?" *Our preexisting state of tension and stress alters the threshold at which a given stimulus is appraised by the amygdala as a threat.*

So, too, does prior experience. The amygdala learns: The first time I take Burleigh to the vet, he enters happily. On the second visit he stiffens his legs and resists going in. On the third visit, as I carry his quivering body into the examining room, he pushes against me, trying to escape. Each successive experience imbues the vet's office with a higher threat evaluation by Burleigh's amygdala, and his defense behavior increases in intensity.

The amygdala also adds **associative triggers** to its list of dangerous stimuli. Just as Pavlov's dog learned to salivate not only at the sight of its dish but at the sound of the bell ringing, the amygdala learns to associate danger with harmless stimuli that occur in close proximity to threatening events. After a series of visits to the vet, I walk into the kitchen one day with an open bottle of rubbing alcohol in my hand. Associating this with his veterinary experiences, Burleigh skulks out of the room.

Let me return to Jim. At my request, he sings a note. It sounds good. But in the next moment his brain hears his sound. Experience has taught him that singing can injure his vocal mechanism. His amygdala responds in an instant, triggering the activation of sympathetic and motor nerves. Now muscles tighten in defense reaction, including the muscles of his vocal mechanism. These tiny muscles no longer coordinate their action with the delicate precision of a moment before and the quality of his sound is diminished. Jim's doctor is at one level correct. The tissues of his vocal folds have healed. However, Jim will not be fully recovered until he can prevent its aftermath, his now habitual fear reaction to the sound of his own voice. *Our preexisting state alters the amygdala's threshold for firing, and experience teaches it to interpret more and more stimuli as threatening. It also assigns its threat evaluation to harmless stimuli that it has learned to associate with danger, acquiring an ever-larger vocabulary of fear.*

THE SHRINKING WORLD OF PAIN

Ed is in his late thirties. He has a slim build, short, curly blond hair, blue eyes, and a nice smile. Ed also has fibromyalgia, a perplexing condition that physicians do not fully understand. The term refers to chronic, unexplained muscle pain and fatigue. The diagnosis recognizes a characteristic group of symptoms; it does not identify their cause. Ed tells me he has had fibromyalgia for several years and has pain throughout his body, especially in his arms and neck. When I question him about his history, he provides a long list of activities and substances (associative triggers) that he believes cause his pain: synthetic fabrics, cold, noise, caffeine, dairy products and many other foods, the computer, driving the car.

He adds that he does not work, seldom goes anywhere, and avoids using his arms. This otherwise healthy and bright young man lives a diminished life. He sits in the chair as I lift his arm, gently supporting it as I seek to lengthen his muscles. Although slender, Ed's arm feels heavy and inert, as if the communication cables have been cut. There is no feeling of connection between an enlivening thought and an alert, responsive musculature. After the lesson he asks my opinion of his problem. I begin by questioning him closely about his activities. Then I ask him why he avoids using his arms.

"Well, for example," he answers, "several days ago I had to drive to an appointment an hour from home. The next day I had a lot of pain in my arms. I had to rest for two days doing absolutely nothing until the pain went away."

"But Ed," I begin slowly, knowing that my remarks will challenge his belief about his condition and how he is handling it, "You have very little muscle mass in your arms. You've curtailed your activity so much that you've stopped using your arms almost completely. As a result, your muscles are withering away. You need to use them more. This may cause you discomfort at first, but I can teach you to do this with a minimum of strain as you regain your strength."

Ed interrupts. "I can't do that. When I use my arms they hurt.

That means I shouldn't use them, right?" Ed has worded the last sentence as a question, but by the tone in his voice I know he isn't asking my opinion. He is telling me what he believes is a fact.

"Actually, pain is a complex business. It doesn't always mean what we think it does. A big pain doesn't always mean a serious problem. A small pain doesn't always mean an insignificant problem. And we don't always know what causes pain. Pain in your muscles doesn't always mean you should stop using them. If we could take a biopsy of your muscle tissue and put it under a microscope, we wouldn't see anything abnormal. Doctors don't really know why patients with fibromyalgia feel pain. You don't have an obvious injury or some type of internal damage.

"We do know it's bad for your muscles not to be used. In fact it may be worse for you than moving and having some pain. You need to build strength. We will proceed slowly and you may have some initial discomfort, but we can work together to develop a system that lets you resume a wider range of activity."

As I am speaking, Ed's expression grows stern. It is clear he is not pleased by what I have said. (A threat.) He stands up abruptly and says he will think about it. I tell him that is fine; he must make whatever decision he feels is best. We are both silent as he walks out of the room and puts on his coat. Ed departs with the briefest goodbye and does not look me in the eye. (*Withdrawal.*)

Neurochemical Response and Stereotyped Defense Behavior

Scientists have learned that the amygdala stimulates glands to produce what are known as *stress hormones* (such as adrenaline and cortisol). In the short term, these help the body cope with pain, inflammation, and injury, but if their production is sustained over a long period due to chronic activation of the amygdala, they produce an array of secondary harmful effects. Studies have linked them to impaired memory and poor decision making, high blood pressure, a weakened immune system, changes in brain chemistry, heart disease, and arthritis.

Chronic conditions such as fibromyalgia are a chicken-and-egg sort of problem. It is hard to know what comes first. Ed's chief complaint is pain. Pain triggers the amygdala to produce stress hormones.

These hormones alter his physiology. In time this lowers the amygdala's threshold, so that less and less pain is required to trigger more and more defense response, as his amygdala in turn produces more stress hormones.[1] Studies have also shown that chronic pain alters the **somatosensory cortex**, so that the brain learns to interpret a wide assortment of bodily sensations as painful.

Ed has also amassed a large number of associative triggers that his amygdala links to danger. Over time this list grows longer, but he does not question his belief that these, too, are harmful and must be guarded against. As Ed recites his list, he does so with gravity, lowering his voice, dropping his head, and shrinking inward as he scans the room for dangerous items.

Whatever its cause, chronic activation of the amygdala and its accompanying overproduction of stress hormones means we are living in the middle of a toxic waste site—ourselves.

Once our worried thoughts are sent on to the amygdala, which generates neurochemical change that triggers the sympathetic and locomotor systems, now, as night must follow day, we must act. The four defense behaviors of vertebrates are withdrawal, freeze, attack, and submit. These are distinct strategies, but they may occur in varying combinations and sequences. They may also be so slight as to constitute nothing more than a drop of our gaze, a hunch of the neck and downward pull on the head, a nervous laugh, a moment's loss of attention.

It is seldom noted that defense is the province of our locomotor system, but without muscles, nerves, bones, and joints we could not withdraw, freeze, attack, or submit. In the short term, the sudden use of our locomotor system for defense (perhaps to run away from an attacking dog) is fine. But living for years with the compounding experiences of threat—internal and external, real and imagined—these structures suffer wear and tear. Sustained for months and years, the amygdala's labors create maladaptive change in muscle activity that hampers how we move. Ed's chronic withdrawal is at least partly responsible for his muscle pain. And recall Jim's muted voice, Joan's immobility, and Burleigh's awkward run.

Such maladaptive locomotor patterns also send their particular sensory stamp back to the brain. By means that are not fully understood, this input gradually produces a faulty conception of the body within the mind itself. Some researchers have termed this phenomena "learning-induced representational catastrophe."[2] Alexander called it **faulty sensory appreciation**. If our physical malcoordination and its accompanying sensory distortion in the brain is repeated long enough, it becomes a fixed behavioral loop, over which we have little control and even less awareness.

A student comes to me complaining of a sharp pain in her lower leg. She tells me that she broke her fibula (a bone in the lower leg) almost two years before. Watching her walk, I see the subtle, telltale imbalance of a limp, a movement pattern she learned in order to compensate for the painful injury. Her leg is now healed, but her limp has become intrinsic to her gait. Every time she takes a step, her brain instructs her body to produce this faulty locomotor pattern. It has failed to correct this compensatory movement when it is no longer needed. Our brain is quick to learn new locomotor patterns in response to threatening or painful stimuli but fails to shed these learned behaviors to restore us to a more balanced coordination when we recover. The original injury has led to a secondary injury within the mind itself, a distorted self-perception that now governs how she moves. This is much harder to identify and more difficult to understand.

My student tells me that her leg still hurts. She insists it is because she is not fully healed. Her belief, which is not correct, further reinforces her defense behavior—limping. She is unaware of this distortion in her walk. When I point it out to her, and explain that this is putting undue strain on muscles and tendons, which probably explains why she is still having pain, she does not believe me. Her way of walking feels normal to her. It is only the pain she feels that she considers to be a problem.

Our stereotyped defense behaviors are played out through the instrument of our psycholocomotor system, but chronic fear and injury create a system that is badly out of tune and difficult to play. They also create a distortion in the mind's perception of how we move and how we are, and this faulty self-perception propels us into further misuse.

For social animals such as humans, our locomotor system offers another type of defense behavior that is often overlooked—the movements of our body communicate our defense strategy to others. Joan's compressed pose is a message for me. ("I feel really bad.")

Burleigh's lowered neck and drooping tail and the act of lying down and rolling over is a message for the other dog. ("I'm weak; it isn't necessary to hurt me, I don't plan to attack.") The other dog's curled lip and deep growl speaks a defensive message as well. ("I'm strong. Better not mess with me or I'll let you have it.")

The remarkable control we can exert over our many facial muscles gives us a subtle skill for defensive messaging. Shadings of attack (Illustration 8-1), withdrawal (Illustration 8-2), freeze (Illustration 8-3), and submit (Illustration 8-4) are evident on the countenances of all you meet, if you observe closely.

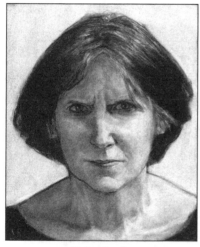

8-1. Attack

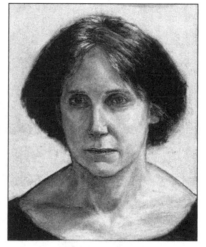

8-2. Withdraw

The four faces of fear. Notice the subtle differences in eye focus and eye position, the differences in expression around the mouth and jaw, and the different wrinkle patterns in the forehead.

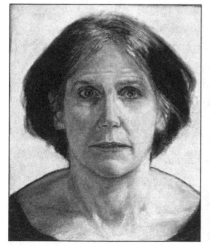

8-3. Freeze

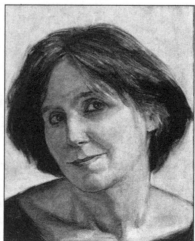

8-4. Submit

Such expressions may take the form of a glimmer of surprise as an eyebrow lifts and lips part; a shadow of downward pull around the lower lip and chin; a brief clench of jaw muscles; a fixed stare. Ineffectual? Most of us can remember a stern expression on the face of a parent or teacher that made us lose our resolve, changing the course of our behavior.

From the standpoint of survival among animals whose own kind may attack them, it is more important to communicate our defense strategy to others than to be able to recognize it in ourselves. Not surprisingly, studies have shown that most of us are highly skilled at reading the subtle facial and postural cues of our species, but as any therapist will attest, oddly slow to perceive our own defense behavior and facial cues.

Over decades, this defensive messaging becomes increasingly fixed. The once neutral, open expression of the child's face becomes etched with unconscious expressions of defense.

There is another category of defense behavior worth noting. This is the change that chronic threat produces in mental alertness. Intriguingly, either end of the alertness spectrum can indicate a threat response. At one end are those who become hyper alert. Such people are highly sensitive to the smallest events, both around them and within themselves, perpetually vigilant for signs of threat and quick to overreact. Although this may give a slight defensive edge under rare circumstances, it causes many other problems.

At the other end of the spectrum are those who are easily distracted and oblivious to events around them. They seem not fully awake and sometimes stubbornly unwilling to face a problem. Not perceiving the effects of their actions or the meaning of other people's behavior, their defense seems to be, "I will deal with this best by not noticing it." This offers an occasional advantage also. Slow to behave defensively, such individuals are less likely to threaten others. But there is a large price to be paid for obliviousness.

Whether hyper- or hypoalert, chronic activation of the amygdala produces maladaptive change in the mind's level of alertness.

Bodily Sensation

Let me recap the first tier of our defense: stimulus, appraisal, neurochemical change, stereotyped behavior, and bodily sensation.

These constitute the essential underpinnings of our defense system, do not require conscious awareness, and are common to vertebrates. The second tier: naming the feeling, creating a self-story, and conscious choice, are largely the province of humans. Further, this second tier depends increasingly on our capacity to be aware of bodily sensation. Our sixth sense could be seen as the link between these two tiers, enabling us to move along a continuum—from unconscious biological processing and stereotyped defense behavior to ever-greater conscious awareness of our inner world, better understanding of our thoughts and behaviors, and greater conscious choice.

In sum, bodily sensation plays a dual role. Since bodily sensations bring us self-awareness, this is the source of our potential for greater choice and control over our behavior. But since this operates within us automatically, it never loses its power to trigger our amygdala, refueling our stereotyped behaviors.

For example, our brain's interpretation of sensory feedback (i.e., feelings, both physical and emotional) can be wrong. We can become so accustomed to the sensory stamp of our defensive behavior that we fail to feel it. As a result, we fail to recognize that our amygdala has perceived a stimulus as a threat, that we are experiencing the neurochemical changes of a threatened organism, and that self-defense is the motivating force beneath our actions. *By blocking out, or becoming habituated to the feelings of our defense behaviors, we fail to recognize that we are in a state of threat.*

We can misjudge our felt experience. I have had students who mistook the sensation of a muscle tensing for that of a muscle relaxing. Jim confuses the feeling of strain in his throat for the cause of his injury rather than the symptom of his fear. Joan misinterprets the pleasurable sensations of her massage treatment as the cause of panic attacks, and so decides to discontinue them. *By misjudging our feelings, we may overlook or mistake the cause of our symptoms. We may also misjudge the efficacy or appropriateness of a treatment.*

We can put our attention on the wrong sensation. We may focus on a pain in our knee, for example, while failing to feel that we are standing on one leg in a way that creates imbalance on the joint and surrounding tissues. Or we may focus on a physical or psychic pain to such an extent that our mind learns to exaggerate the perception of this feeling, while blocking out or diminishing our awareness of other sensations. *By overfocusing our attention on pain or other types of sensations, we inadvertently magnify our perception of them, and so may fail to notice other important sensory inputs.*

We can recall our feelings for long periods of time, as our mind summons the sensation of remembered sensation. If you have spent several days on a boat, you have probably noticed that you felt the familiar feeling of rocking for days afterward. Contrary to popular myth, this sensation is not caused by the ongoing movement of fluid in the inner ear, since this fluid stops moving shortly after you return to land. The feeling of rocking is simply a remembered feeling. *People who have suffered from extreme pain—physical or mental—yearn to vanquish this from their memory. Somatic memory enables us to experience our trauma over and over and over again.*

We can mistakenly assume that any unpleasant feeling means danger and should be avoided. Our Western culture is widely imbued with the simplistic idea that all uncomfortable sensations are bad and all pleasing sensations are good. *As a culture we largely neglect to teach our young that it is possible to tolerate reasonable levels of discomfort without reacting in defense. In some cases this skill is an appropriate behavioral choice, but it needs to be practiced.*

Finally, as we will see next, we can focus our attention on the sensations that are produced *after* we are triggered into a threat behavior (pounding heart and shaking muscles) while failing to notice the sensations that trigger it.

9

Anxiety and Performance

Experience is not what happens to you;
it's what you do with what happens to you.
—ALDOUS HUXLEY

BRUCE, PART ONE

BRUCE IS A talented young pianist of medium height and build, with wavy brown hair and a boyish face. He tells me during his first lesson that he could never have a professional career because of his performance anxiety.

"My muscles get shaky. I feel my heart pounding in my chest. It's hard to breathe. I can't concentrate. I get dizzy. I know I can't do anything about this," he adds, "but I thought I'd give the Alexander Technique a try. What the heck."

Bruce has now had ten lessons. Today is the first time I have asked him to play the piano. As I listen, I notice his skill and facility at the keyboard. His locomotor coordination presents some problems, but nothing too out of the ordinary.

Occasionally Bruce makes a mistake. I watch closely. Each time a finger misses a note his expression becomes more determined. He purses his lips as a bulge of muscle presses outward along his jaw. His neck muscles tighten also, pulling his head back and raising his

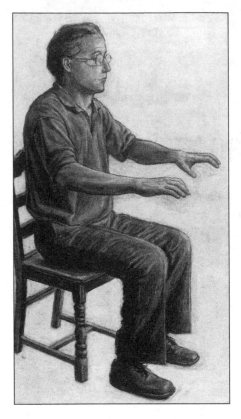

shoulders. This tension spreads into his arms and hands. He holds his breath (Illustration 9–1).

After a while I ask him to stop. Bruce turns his head to look at me, exasperation etched on his face. "Now you see what I'm talking about. I should have played this perfectly. I've practiced it a lot. But when I play in front of people I make stupid mistakes. My fingers don't do what I want. All I have to do is imagine someone watching me and I get these weird sensations in my body and I mess up.

"I've had this problem as far back as I can remember. It's getting worse. I had a judgmental teacher when I was young. I think that's what caused it. I couldn't ever play well enough to satisfy her."

"What things have you tried for this?"

"I did yoga and learned breathing exercises. I exercise on the day of performance. Sometimes I take beta-blockers. They help, but they make me feel disconnected. I can't get as passionate about the music."

Pointing to one of the passages that gave him difficulty, I ask Bruce to play it again. He has the same problem.

9–1. Bruce sitting with his arms poised for playing the piano. His shoulders are raised and his neck muscles are tight, pulling his head down toward his body. The muscles of his arms are tense and his fingers are stiff.

"What were you thinking about while you were playing? Can you say?"

"I started thinking about that difficult section and hoping I wouldn't make a mistake. I was thinking about it and trying to get ready for it. I had a teacher who told me to read ahead in the music and prepare myself in my mind for the hard parts."

"Were you thinking anything else?"

"I was aware of you watching me, wondering what you'd think."

"Why don't you play it again? See if there's anything else that catches your attention. Take time to observe yourself and collect information about what's happening within you, mentally and physically, as you play." Bruce plays again and then stops.

"Notice anything?"

"I got more tense just before those tough measures."

"When you say that you got tense, what do you mean? How did you recognize that?"

Bruce plays the passage again, stops, and then turns to me.

"I felt some tightening in my neck and throat before I got to those hard parts."

"What happened first? Was it thinking about the difficult parts or feeling the tension?"

"Actually, it was the thought. A split second later I felt the tension. But it was just the briefest flash of a thought. I don't know if I could call it a thought exactly, but something changed in my mind. Then tension seemed to well up almost instantaneously. I felt it in my neck. It's hard to describe. If I hadn't had these lessons, I'd never have noticed."

"You're gathering important information, Bruce. Try another passage.

Bruce plays a new section. Again he has difficulty. Shortly afterward he stops and turns to me. This time his expression is not as serious. Instead he looks almost eager.

"I was playing okay. Then I started thinking about that hard passage and trying to get ready for it. Immediately I felt that tension in my neck again, then my fingers stiffened and I missed the notes. But it happened so fast."

"That's terrific, Bruce. You're learning to recognize the moment that your thinking triggers you into fear. This is what leads to those weird sensations in your body that you call performance anxiety. If we can get a better handle on when it begins, we have something we can work with. Play again."

As Bruce plays, I notice him increasing his tempo. Shortly afterward he makes another mistake. He stops playing immediately and turns to me. "You know what happened this time?"

"What?"

"I was playing well. Then I had the thought that I was playing well, and I got tense and messed up. I actually got more anxious and tense because I was thinking about how well I was playing!"

"This is another great observation, Bruce. You're learning to notice the connection between when your thinking goes off track—and even thoughts like the fact that you're playing well can trigger fear—and the reaction this creates in your body that interferes with your coordination, physically and mentally. It's the whole of you that's affected by how you think, not just your fingers. It triggers neurochemical changes that interfere with your muscular coordination as you play, and make it harder for you to keep your mind on what you're doing. In turn, you're more likely to think in a way that causes you to trigger more fear. It's a vicious circle."

Bruce looks out the window. Without turning his head he says, "I've been causing this problem in myself, haven't I?"

Naming the Feeling, Creating a Self-Story

Our mind gathers our bodily sensations into a *self-construct*—a concept of a self that is "me." This can be likened to a mirror in the mind, which forms an image from bodily inputs that is reflected onto our **awareness**. When this self-construct is combined with our capacity to think in words, now we can speak about this self, reflect on it, and observe its behavior. Our capacity to think with words can be likened to a second mirror, positioned facing the first. Language enables us to reflect on the reflection. Now the self-image bounces back and forth, from one to the other, virtually without end: We can reflect on our reflection. We can see our selves in the act of seeing our selves. We can identify a particular feeling as *mine*, choose to focus our attention on it, describe it, and think about it again and again. How we think about our feelings also generates more feelings.

More important, the mind infers *meaning* from these self-reflections: "I'm feeling out of sorts. Maybe it's from that phone conversation I had last night."

We also make decisions based on this meaning: "It must be because of that phone conversation. I'm not going to talk on the phone at night anymore."

Together, our powers of self-construction and self-reflection are a formidable combination. They give us an enormous edge over other animals. But unbeknownst to us, our mirrors can become flawed. Our sensory awareness can be incomplete and inaccurate. The meaning we ascribe to a feeling is only a best guess. And words are symbols, approximations of our state of being. Over the course of our lives our mirrors become more and more warped, creating and reflecting images of our selves to our selves that are ever more distorted.

Since we have a vast supply of words with which to name and describe our feelings, our choice of words is often inconsistent. It may also be misleading. Today you might say that you feel worried, but next week the same sensation might cause you to say you feel tired or depressed. The feelings that you call anxiety someone else might call exhilaration. *We do not use the same words, reliably and consistently over time, to identify a particular feeling—either to ourselves or in communication with others. And two people may name the same feeling differently.*

The rich vocabulary of our inner life of sensation—especially the feelings we speak of as emotions—leads us to believe that there are as many emotions as there are words to describe them. We think of our feelings/emotions as if they were problems in themselves to be discussed, analyzed, and managed like misbehaving children. But feelings/emotions are not words, things, or beings. As we experience them through our awareness, they are only gossamer glimpses of the continually changing state of our organism. Words are a further reflection of this image, twice removed from the actual moment when our amygdala is activated into defense, a mechanism of which we have no conscious perception. *The sensations of our emotions, specifically fear and anxiety, are an unintended consequence—the shimmering aftereffect of the amygdala's activation—that reverberate upward to our awareness like waves after a pebble breaks the water's surface.*

In the case of uncomfortable or painful feelings we often seek a diagnosis, using more words to name our condition: Joan has panic attacks; Jim has a vocal problem; Ed has fibromyalgia; Bruce has performance anxiety. But diagnosis connotes disease and all that this implies. We assume that some type of medical treatment is required and that only a physician or medical professional can help us. Although many of the problems and conditions created by our self-driven anxiety are painful, and can seriously undermine our health and create behaviors over which we have little control, they are not really medical problems. There is no invading microorganism. There is no sudden trauma. There is no congenital disorder. *There is only an endlessly self-reflecting and distorted image in our minds, which holds surprising power to influence our behavior and shape our inner life.*

We also use words to create self-stories, sometimes of amazing complexity, in a further effort to make sense of the multitude of bodily sensations we experience, especially disturbing sensations such as fear and anxiety. Our stories lend a sense of cohesion to disparate feelings, but we fail to recognize that they are a straw house built of partial understanding, distortion, and guesswork. They are a skewed frame of reference, yet they become ever more solidified in our mind as beliefs that hold us in their grip, limiting our thinking and narrowing our behavioral choices. These beliefs are like a snapshot of the reflection in the mirror, a picture that we carry forever in our mind as true—how it is and how it must be. Because of these beliefs, we not only confine ourselves to living in a single room, we believe ourselves to be locked in.

Bruce has performance anxiety, he says, because of a judgmental teacher when he was young. Believing that his performance anxiety is caused by events in the past, and since these events cannot possibly be changed, it follows in his mind that his performance anxiety is immutable. Ed does not know why he has fibromyalgia. No one does. But he has created a complex story explaining why he must avoid each of many associative triggers. Seeking whenever possible to avoid these triggers, he lives in a smaller and smaller world, self-filtering any new experiences that might provide him an opportunity to discover the flaw in his belief. Ed believes he is locked in his room, and never tries the door.

Our beliefs not only limit our thinking, they steer us in the wrong direction. We may pay more attention to our beliefs than to what is actually happening within us and around us in the present moment. We become oblivious to important information that might disprove our beliefs. Only feelings and experiences that really hit us over the head get our attention. The subtle cues of back pain, for example, do not jibe with our belief that we are strong and healthy. It is easy to ignore these feelings, at least until the day that we bend over, feel a sudden shooting pain, and cannot stand up. We also fail to notice the subtle inner dialogue of beliefs that we recite to ourselves, triggering our fear, and notice instead only the sensations of anxiety that are the result.

Bruce's mind is focused on his feelings of performance anxiety (beating heart, queasy stomach, shaking hands), but these are the byproducts of his amygdala's activity. Over time he has become increasingly *reactive,* ever more fearful of his feelings of fear. Bruce can tell me his diagnosis and describe his anxiety in detail. He can recount his self-story, which has become a strongly held belief about his condition and what has caused it. But he has not noticed that his thoughts and beliefs are fueling his fear.

In sum, the dual mirrors of self-perception and self-reflection are by nature imprecise, and may become increasingly warped over time through acquired patterns of poor locomotor coordination, as well as through further pain, injury, and other traumatic experiences. This incomplete and skewed self-image is further distorted by what we say to ourselves about ourselves (and what we tell others) and becomes ever more embedded in our mind as belief, which we regard as truth.

Conscious Choice

Self-awareness and self-reflection can be used to give us another option. We can think about our behavior and consciously choose another. We do not have conscious choice over the amygdala's decision to appraise a given stimulus as a threat; once this happens, we are propelled into behaviors of defense. But we can become aware of our overt behavior and decide to select another. *We have some conscious choice.*

After Ed left his lesson, I did not think it likely he would call again. I knew I was telling him something that challenged the story he had created to support his defense behavior. He responded as I expected, in defense of his defense. But a year later I picked up the phone one day, and Ed was on the line asking for another appointment. I asked him how he had been.

"After I saw you I gave some thought to what you said. I started seeing a physical therapist. I told him I wanted to strengthen my arms. He gave me some exercises. At my appointment last week, he told me I've significantly increased my strength since last year." There was an unmistakable tone of pride in Ed's voice as he added, "I thought it was a good time to come back and see you."

The good news is that through conscious choice we can change our defense behavior. Admittedly this is difficult when we are under the duress of a fear reaction, but sometimes we can stop, reframe our situation in our mind, and make a different choice.

The bad news is that this may only amount to swapping one defense behavior for another, when neither is particularly beneficial. Further, it does not alter the driving force behind our defense behavior, which as we have seen often comes from our own barely conscious thoughts and feelings. Selecting a different behavioral response is an option and may be helpful, but it is not entirely a solution. It only gives us the opportunity to alter our behavior at the far end, after we have been triggered into defense.

Is there a way of changing what happens at the beginning? Can we learn to stop the stream of stimuli we send to our amygdala, thus lowering its activity?

Through his lessons Bruce is learning to recognize the feelings and thoughts that trigger him into his fear reaction. He is learning to recognize that the mirrors in his mind and the beliefs he has formed from them are distorted. Gradually he is developing more accurate self-perception. He can perceive that he is causing his problem and when he is doing it. Armed with these insights, he is ready to repair the mirrors. He is ready to learn the skills of self-correction.

10

Attention, Awareness, and Conscious Inhibition

To get what you want, stop doing what isn't working.

—EARL WARREN

BRUCE, PART TWO

"Bruce, I'D LIKE you to try something. This time as you play, whenever you notice either your mind wandering—thinking about me, the difficult parts, or how well you're doing—or if you simply notice a feeling of tension in your neck and shoulders, I'd like you to think to yourself, *I'm not playing the piano.*"

Bruce's head swivels toward me as he raises his eyebrows. "You want me to think, *I'm NOT playing the piano*? What's the point of that?"

"Yes, I know this sounds strange, but bear with me for a moment. When you play those hard passages you feel tense and anxious, right?"

Bruce nods his head.

"How about when you walk down the street? Do you have performance anxiety then?"

Bruce's face expands into a grin. "Of course not."

"Why not?"

"Because I'm not playing the piano!" he answers, exasperated.

"That's right. If there's no piano, there's nothing to fear. What about when you simply sit at the piano with your hands in your lap?"

Bruce turns to face his music again and puts his hands on his thighs. He is silent. After a moment he turns back to me. "I'm feeling more anxious," he says softly.

"This is my point. The piano is a trigger. You aren't aware of it, but just by sitting at the piano in a sense your brain is already thinking, *I'm going to play the piano*. All you have to do is sit at the piano and at some level your mind knows what you're going to do as well as what might happen."

"Make a mistake?" Bruce says, finishing my thought.

"You've got it. Your mind has learned to associate making mistakes with the piano itself. You don't have to touch the keys. Seeing the piano is a stimulus that your brain perceives as a threat, triggering an array of fear reactions, some of which are fed back to you as certain sensations. Then you recognize these and say you feel anxious.

"Let's shift gears and try a slightly different experiment. I want you to sit facing the piano with your hands in your lap. Notice those feelings of anxiety, but tell yourself you're not playing the piano. Silently repeat that thought in your mind a number of times and notice if the feelings of anxiety lessen. If they do, put your hands on the keys and notice what happens when you do that."

Bruce sits quietly at the keyboard, hands in his lap. He does not move or speak for several minutes. Then he puts his hands on the piano.

"Well?" I ask, as he turns to look at me.

"As I was sitting I was feeling a little anxious. Not a lot. I told myself I wasn't playing so there wasn't anything to worry about, and gradually I began to feel better. Then I put my hands on the keys."

"What did you notice?"

"My heart started pounding."

"Okay, that's great. So seeing the piano is a trigger, and putting your hands on the keys is an even more powerful trigger. This is great. You're learning and observing a lot. Do the same thing again. Sit with your hands in your lap and think of not playing until you feel calmer. Then put your hands on the keys and notice your reaction, and say to yourself again, 'I'm not playing the piano.' Leave your hands on the keys and repeat this thought for several minutes."

Bruce faces the keyboard, his hands in his lap as before. After several minutes he puts his hands on the keys. He leaves them there for several minutes and then he puts his hands back in his lap.

"What about this time?" I ask.

"When I first put them on the keyboard I got really tense. I felt my head pull back and down and my neck stiffen. My arms felt heavier. It was hard to breathe. Then I told myself I wasn't playing. After a while my body eased up. My arms felt lighter. I was breathing better."

"That's terrific, Bruce. You're learning to change how you are thinking and that is changing the tension level in your muscles, as well as your anxiety.

"Now this time, begin by repeating the first two steps: Think of not playing while your hands are in your lap. When you are calmer, put your hands on the keys and think of not playing as you rest your fingers on the keyboard. When you're feeling better, go ahead and play, but as you're playing, whenever you notice yourself reverting back to the old thoughts or tensions, stop playing and just leave your hands on the keys. Don't take them off the piano. Leave them on the keys and think, *I'm not playing*. When you are feeling calmer, resume playing again.

"I want you to stop playing each time you notice your thoughts wandering, your muscles tensing, or those feelings of anxiety creeping in. Even if it's only a note or two after you've just resumed playing. Each time you stop take as much time as you need. There's no hurry to begin again. Think of not playing. Wait until those feelings of anxiety fade away completely. Got it?"

Bruce nods, places his hands on his lap, waits, and then puts them on the keyboard. He stops again for a short while and then begins playing. Soon afterward he stops. After a minute he begins again. Then he stops once more, waits silently, and begins again. He continues playing, stopping and starting, for about ten minutes. Gradually his neck

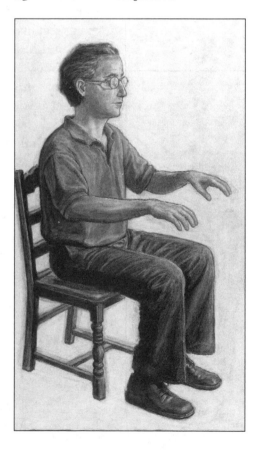

10-1. Bruce sitting with his arms poised for playing while he thinks of not playing. There is less tension in his neck muscles, which allows his neck to lengthen upward and his head to move forward and up. His shoulders are wide apart, his arms are looser, and his fingers have lengthened.

and shoulder tension eases (see Illustration 10-1). He stops less often, his tempo evens, and he makes fewer mistakes.

When he takes his hands off the keyboard I ask, "What did you notice this time?"

Bruce does not answer immediately, but continues looking intently at the keys. "That was really interesting," he says slowly. "At first I had to stop a lot but it got better toward the end. My mind didn't wander as much. I was worrying less. And I felt better. This is making me realize how often I lose my attention when I'm playing. One moment it's there, the next moment it's somewhere else. I don't think I'm really thinking about the music that clearly, especially since I know this piece so well. As soon as my thinking shifts and goes off track, something changes physically. I can sense that now. Somehow it makes the muscles in my neck and arms tighten, and I miss notes.

"When I stopped, and thought of not playing as you asked, then I just seemed to get calm again, and my mind got back on track. I didn't feel like a runaway train. Each time I began again, my playing was a little better. My thinking was clearer. My fingers were more fluid."

"That's great, Bruce. You're making important connections to yourself as you are playing. It's not just a matter of making the fingers hit the right keys at the right time. You have to connect with yourself—mind and body—thoughts, movements, and feelings.

"This time you're going to begin by doing the same thing. Stop playing when you notice the tension building or your thoughts wandering. Just leave your hands on the keyboard and think of not playing. Then when you're feeling calmer, continue thinking to yourself that you're *not* playing as you resume playing."

"That doesn't make sense," Bruce interrupts. "How can I play while I'm telling myself I'm not playing?"

"I know this sounds nonsensical, but it's easy. You can play as you think to yourself that a hard passage is coming up and that you might make a mistake, right?"

"Yeah."

"Now you're going to play as you think to yourself that you're not playing."

Bruce shakes his head, but turns back to the keyboard and places his hands in his lap. After a minute he puts his hands on the keys and stops. After several more minutes he begins to play. Periodically he stops again, leaves his hands on the keys, and then resumes. After about ten minutes of stopping frequently, he continues playing uninterrupted. I notice now that his fingers are more fluid and confident. His tempo is even. There is a new energy in his sound, as if he is poised on the top of a wave, feeling the wave's power surging beneath him and confidently drawing from it, letting it carry him forward while he pushes against it. There is a quality of connection and strength in Bruce's playing, yet he looks relaxed and calm.

After he finishes the piece, Bruce turns toward me. His expression shows his pleasure. "That felt great!"

I meet his smile with my own. "Bruce, that time your playing gave me goose bumps."

Bruce looks back at the keyboard, pulled by the memory of this new sense of power and connection within himself. Still smiling, he says, "If I keep practicing this way I think I can turn this thing around."

Conscious Inhibition

The process I am engaging in with Bruce is designed to help him notice subtle bodily sensations and shifts in his mental attention that he has not perceived before. He is learning to identify the **initiating triggers** of his fear. The earlier lessons have aided this process by teaching him to restore a better overall locomotor coordination as he plays. He has been learning to shed muscle tension that marred his ability to perceive what he was doing. Now that he can more readily recognize his initiating triggers, I have asked him to stop whenever he notices this happening and insert a new stimulus—*the thought of not playing*.

Bruce reacted to this idea just as most students do. "What? Why would I do that? That doesn't make any sense," they invariably say.

To think of not doing something sounds strange. To think of not doing an activity while we are actually doing it sounds impossible. Yet when Bruce tried it, he experienced surprising changes. He found himself feeling calmer, less distracted, and less tense. His fingers moved more smoothly and he made fewer mistakes.

Bruce is learning to think in a manner that is, essentially, canceling his message to his amygdala: "I'm not playing, so there's no need to send the alarm." By changing what he is thinking in this way, he is changing how his mind is behaving. Since his thoughts can stimulate his amygdala to produce anxiety, they can also lessen or prevent this stimulus, and so indirectly alter his neurochemistry and defense reaction. This is not conscious choice but *conscious inhibition*. *It is the ability to cease unwanted activity in the organism at a neurological level through conscious thought, which in turn changes the organism's activity at a larger, behavioral level.*

In part 3, we will explore conscious inhibition, beginning with a story about my own exploration into this vital skill. I will also draw from recent research in neuroscience to help us better understand inhibition's physiological basis. Then we will look at this skill in action: Chapter 13 recounts the story of how I taught my ten-year-old son conscious inhibition to help him keep his eyes on the ball to improve his batting. We will return to Erin in her lessons as she is learning to inhibit to reduce muscle tension and improve the functioning of her locomotor system. Finally, in the self-experiments at the end of part 3, you will have an opportunity to learn this vital skill.

HOW DO YOU THINK?

THE MIND CHANGES EVERYTHING

A Fine Day in London with Nothing to Feel

O day and night, but this is wondrous strange!
—WILLIAM SHAKESPEARE

ONE BEAUTIFUL JULY afternoon I arrived at 18 Lansdowne Road in London for an Alexander lesson with Walter Carrington, a world-renowned teacher of the Technique. He ushered me into his teaching room. I recall standing in front of the chair, alternately eyeing the familiar objects around me and gazing out the window as his hands spilled across my back and shoulders. We chatted the entire lesson as Carrington's hands gently urged my muscles to give up their hold on my bones. Moving me in and out of the chair, up and down, again and again, he was reshaping me in ways that I could only dimly comprehend. I noticed my ribs moving more readily, rhythmically drawing my breath in then powerfully releasing it out again. My back was fanning open. My feet were releasing their clamp on the floor.

What was keeping me upright?

All the while some mysterious infusion seemed to shift my mind from its typically harried, crowded state into quiet, open space.

None of this seemed particularly unusual. It was just another fine lesson from my teacher that produced the familiar experience of becoming looser and lighter as if shedding a decade from my sinews. My first awareness that something was distinctly other-than-usual occurred hours later in the middle of the night. I awoke and felt the muscles in my lower back—my former dancer's narrow, steel-cabled back—letting loose. It felt as though I was peeling open and spreading, then falling, weightless. Since I had never felt anything like this before, I tried staying awake to experience the sensation a bit longer. But sleep soon arrived, followed too quickly by the insistent buzz of the alarm.

Rolling over in bed to begin the day, my first conscious thought was that the sensation of release in my muscles was gone. But I had a vague sense that something else was absent as well, as though I had fallen asleep at a large party and wakened to find everyone gone. What was it? I stood up and walked into the bathroom, considering an array of possibilities. Then realization dawned. I was not only missing the sensation of muscular release in my back, I was missing sensation entirely.

Where did my body go?

I glanced quickly in the mirror and grinned from sheer relief as I saw my face reflected back to me. Yet as I did this, there was no answering echo of bodily feeling, telling me I had performed the movement. I was not experiencing a feeling of numbness, but rather of emptiness. When I closed my eyes it seemed as though my lifelong companion, my body, had disappeared. Unsure what to do I began scanning internal systems, like a pilot checking his instruments before takeoff. Vision? That's okay; I can see myself in the mirror. Hearing? I'm aware of the traffic in the street. Thinking? I know who I am, where I am, the date and time. Now what?

"Just keep doing what you usually do," an inner voice suggested. So I dismissed the waves of alarm that were lining up in my mind like soldiers on parade and started downstairs for breakfast. But as I began to walk, I became aware of a strange sense that I was not the one working the controls in myself. Something else within me seemed to be dictating the precise bend of my legs, the counter-balancing swing of my arms, the upward poise of my head on my neck. There was no feeling of pressure on my feet as I stepped. I briefly wondered if my body had been occupied in the middle of the night by some strange alien with a special skill for operating the controls to my body.

Later that day, walking along the London streets, I glanced down to see if my body was still there. I did not know I was moving except by the reassuring sight of buildings disappearing as I passed them. There were a few small sensations like the wind blowing across my face and through my hair, but the internal cues of a body in motion were switched off. I decided to take longer strides than what this alien force within me was prescribing. Sensations suddenly began flooding through me again as "muscles" seemed to spring into action to do the work of moving my "body." I shortened my stride. Immediately some other force seemed to reel me back in and take command, as my physical self all but evaporated from my mind.

It appeared I had a choice: I could decide to take over the controls if I wished and return to my old habits of moving and the bodily sensations that accompanied it. Or I could allow myself to be moved by this other force, remain within the invisible boundary of a previously unknown but marvelous new coordination of myself, and let the layers of feelings fall away. It was not a hard decision. I was fascinated and thrilled by this improbable release from sensation's gusty winds. Without my feelings distracting me, my mood was calm. My mind was alert. It was as if I had been living for years next to a highway, oblivious to the noise of cars speeding by, and then one day moving to the country and discovering silence for the first time. My mental screen was blank. The water was clear.

This strange phenomenon lasted for almost a week and then faded. I did not understand what had happened to me, yet I felt certain that the memory of my experience would return and gradually reveal its meaning. For the present I was satisfied with a simple sense of awe. As I described it to a friend, it was as if I had found an old lamp and, rubbing it, had summoned a genie who presented me with a priceless gift: a glimpse, not of my future, but of a potential within myself I had never known.

I began to appreciate how deeply attached I was to the feeling of my muscles working. My muscle tension reassured me that I existed, created my belief in my need to try harder, told me that I was in fact doing and trying as I believed I should. I could see my error now, the hairline fracture in the struts of my logic. It was all so unnecessary. I had been released not just from my tension but from my belief about its necessity and importance. It was not so much that I thought of myself as different, I tried eagerly to explain to my friend; it was that my *self* was able to think differently.

Over the succeeding months I scanned my mind for answers, hoping to recapture the experience. As I did, long-unanswered questions and worries about my teaching arose as well. Why was I frequently more tired and tense after teaching? Why did I feel a peculiar sense of anxiety as I waited for my students to arrive? I knew my students were learning a lot, but why didn't they magically release from the contact of my hands as I did beneath Carrington's? With each passing day it seemed I was moving further away from my experience in London, not closer to it.

In time I began to see that my lesson with Carrington had enabled me to let go of unnecessary tension as never before. His hands had helped me to achieve a new level of *inhibition* in myself. What else could explain the phenomenal late-night release in my musculature? And the astonishing new ease with which I moved?

With the memory of my London experience shining like a beacon in my mind, it seemed likely that the solution to my questions boiled down to one essential—namely, that I did not understand and practice conscious inhibition well enough. I concluded that this skill held the potential for producing greater physiological and psychological benefits than I had realized. I became determined to unlock its secrets—to learn how to use this skill consciously and consistently, so that I could recreate these marvelous changes for myself.

Discovering the Thinking Mind

We are not what we know,
but what we are willing to learn.
—MARY CATHERINE BATESON

SEARCHING FOR CLUES, I reread Alexander's story of discovery, "Evolution of a Technique."[1] Observing himself in the mirror, he saw that each time he had a thought of speaking his muscles tensed excessively. Then he told himself *not* to speak and his tension melted away. I contrasted Alexander's account with what has been distilled and passed on to succeeding generations of Alexander teachers and students. We say that when we are aware of a stimulus that triggers us to react, inhibition lets us stop and think again. It creates a window in time through which new choices can emerge. It enables us to decide to do something else.

We may decide to go for a walk, for example, but then by inhibiting we may decide not to go and stay home. We may notice our muscles tightening and decide not to tense them. We may notice when an emotional reaction wells up, like an urge to yell at someone perhaps, and then think better of the impulse and take a deep breath instead.

Now I realized that this explanation was insufficient. Alexander did not just *decide* to speak or not to speak. He *thought* of not speaking and, by his own report, he thought this thought over and over again.

I pored over written accounts by Alexander's students of their lessons. Writing in his diary in 1952, Goddard Binkley recalled Alexander emphasizing "how important it is to grasp the principal of **non-doing** [inhibition] . . . [and that he] had racked his brain for a long time over the question of what was the best way to get this across to pupils."[2] Binkley also reported Alexander telling him, "I spent days, months, years practicing inhibition. I had no one standing by my side telling me what not to do. I kept it up, until one day I got up out of my chair without effort. I just shot right up."[3] And on another occasion, "This is the principle of the whole work—not to do something but to think. We redirect our activity by means of thought alone. This principle is the hardest of all to grasp. People just don't see it. Yet we know that it works. It is demonstrable."[4]

If inhibiting were only a matter of deciding to do something else, I thought, surely Alexander would not need to "rack his brains" trying to figure out how to explain it to his students or spend so long practicing it.

Was there something different about the way he thought of not speaking that produced his dramatic vocal recovery? If so, why did his thinking succeed whereas my own seldom did?

I decided to follow Alexander's example. Sitting in a chair I repeated to myself, "I'm not standing up." At first I felt embarrassed. What nonsense was I engaged in? Then I began to feel an inner readiness draining from my muscles—tension I had not realized I was holding until I felt it melt away. My breathing deepened. I felt more balanced and at ease. I had not decided to stop doing a specific thing and then to do something else. I had simply sat, unmoving, thinking my thought of not standing. Was it possible for a thought such as this to produce a physical change—a change that was both beneficial and *unexpected*? I had not decided to make my muscles release. How did it happen?

Muscle activity requires nerve activity, I reasoned, since muscles do not operate without a signal and the signal is sent via nerves and begins in the brain. This meant that by thinking words such as "I'm not standing," I was changing nerve and brain activity. This was a simple line of logic and a small beginning, yet it left me with a sense of unease. I was being pushed off my comfortable perch of certainty like a boulder in a mudslide. I was on unfamiliar ground.

This new ground was neuroscience and recent research into the mind and consciousness. Books by Damasio, Hobson, Ramachandran, Goldberg, and others began to line my shelves. I became fascinated by research on the brain's frontal lobes, especially the **prefrontal cortex**, an area of the brain above the eyes in the front of the skull. Scientists have learned that in evolutionary terms, this is our brain's newest area. It is also the region that develops latest as we grow, not coming fully online until we reach our early twenties.

Significant advances in technology have brought brain-imaging techniques such as functional magnetic resonance imaging (fMRI) and positron emission tomography (PET). These produce pictures of the brain in activity. As subjects are asked to perform a task, precise areas of the brain become redder in color as metabolic activity is increased due to increased blood flow. Other areas shift to green and purple as metabolic activity is decreased, indicating less activity and blood flow. These images enable neuroscientists to link a task that a subject is asked to perform with the area of the brain that is used to perform it. This has helped scientists learn that the prefrontal cortex is like the conductor of the orchestra. It does not play an individual instrument so much as it oversees the activity of the whole.[5]

For example, the prefrontal cortex is vital for performing such tasks as planning and thinking ahead, being aware of our body and what we are doing, regulating our mood and, significantly, *controlling impulses*—that is, inhibiting unwanted, unnecessary, or inappropriate urges, thoughts, and actions as they arise in the mind. It also helps prevent the mind from randomly shifting attention from one stimulus to the next.[6]

Research into behavioral disorders, such as attention deficit disorder (ADD), hyperactivity disorder (HD), or both (ADHD) using brain scans has shown that individuals with these disorders have lower levels of metabolic activity in the prefrontal cortex than normal subjects. This means that such individuals are less able to control impulses such as hyperactivity, emotional outbursts, and mental distraction. Further evidence for the importance of the prefrontal cortex in controlling impulsive behavior has been shown in studies of people who are highly aggressive. Many of these people have suffered frontal lobe damage, often caused by birth trauma or head injury, and their brain scans show a diminished level of activity in the prefrontal cortex.[7]

For those with ADD and ADHD, stimulants such as Ritalin and caffeine can reduce symptoms because they supplement low levels of neurotransmitters such as dopamine and serotonin that boost the metabolic activity of this area of the brain.[8] (Perhaps this explained why I could not balance my checkbook before my morning cup of tea!)

Research on the prefrontal cortex by Hanna Damasio, neuroscientist at the University of Iowa College of Medicine, has produced strikingly different images of brain activity when subjects are asked to think happy thoughts as opposed to depressed, worried, or anxious thoughts. The brain scans of those thinking happy thoughts show an increased metabolic activity in the prefrontal cortex. By contrast, each of the others shows increased activity in lower, subcortical areas of the brain.

An interesting study using brain scan techniques has shown a difference in brain activity between amateur and professional musicians. When the amateurs played their instruments, the motor cortex (for movement) lit up, brightly red, on the images. When the professionals played, the auditory cortex (for sound) jumped into action. It appears that the two groups have learned to use their brains differently as they play. The amateurs focus their mind on the motor activity aspect of their performance, deciding where to put their fingers and how to move them. By contrast, the professionals think about the sounds they want to produce. They are organizing their movements by putting their attention on creating this sound, rather than on doing specific movements in the body.[9]

The implication of this study and others for the essential role that learning plays in determining brain function is striking. It appears that our higher, cortical brain activity is not as strictly determined by the chance of our genetic inheritance as previously thought. Learning plays a key role not just in *what* we think, but also in *how* we think.[10] In the Alexander Technique, we speak of our learned habits of misuse, but in view of recent research, *our physical habits could be more accurately described as outward reflections of an underlying use of ourselves that lies hidden from view—the learned use (or misuse) of the mind itself.*

Armed with these insights it seemed likely that Alexander's instruction to think of not speaking, or not standing, had achieved its notable outcome because, like the professional musicians, his thinking was coordinated in a way that was different from my own. I had assumed that if I simply spoke his verbal instructions to myself the desired response would occur. But if my thought of *non-doing* was not constructed the same as his—if I was using my brain differently— then it followed that the outcome would be different, too.

Further, I reasoned, if those with ADD suffered from reduced inhibitory control due to lower metabolic activity in the prefrontal cortex, could there not also be differences in prefrontal activity in normal individuals? Might this be more common than previously considered? If it was possible to increase the metabolic activity of the prefrontal cortex simply by thinking happy thoughts, as shown in Damasio's study, might it be possible to *consciously* increase the activity level of the prefrontal cortex, and thus improve inhibitory functioning?

As I sorted through this array of information and speculation, I was struck by the coincidence that the prefrontal cortex is located forward and up within the brain itself, and that Alexander had specifically instructed his students to think, "forward and up." Could it be that Alexander's recommendation to think of the head forward and up was the means by which he had increased the activity of his prefrontal cortex, thus enabling him to better inhibit harmful tension that marred the functioning of his vocal mechanism?

How could I find out if my own prefrontal activity was up to par? Could I learn, consciously, to improve its functioning? More to the point, how was I to find the answers to my questions without a highly skilled teacher—or a brain scan—to guide me?

THE ATTIC

One day I was lying on my back on the floor (this is the semisupine position that you explored in section A) thinking to myself not to tighten my neck as Alexander instructed, when I became aware of a subtle quality of dropping downward in myself. Again I thought of not tightening my neck. Again I noticed my eyes dropping down, and a slight pulling sensation in my chest and throat. My breathing became more constricted, and my overall awareness seemed to be drawn inward. It seemed as if I was focusing all my **attention** on the specific part of my body—my neck—that I had just named in my mind.

Why did I do that?

I repeated the instructions. The same downward shift of attention and inward response was triggered.

Was it possible to think of not tensing my neck without producing this reaction?

Since I did not know if this was inevitable, or what I could do to prevent it, I decided just to continue paying close attention to myself as I thought Alexander's instructions. Soon my awareness of the downward pull and inward focus became distinct. The reaction was small but unmistakable.

Why hadn't I noticed this before?

Several weeks later, I recalled the odd coincidence that Alexander advised thinking of the head *forward and up,* and that the prefrontal cortex is located forward and up within the brain itself. I began wondering what a scan of my brain would show if I thought of my head forward and up on the top of my neck.

Could such a thought possibly have an effect on my prefrontal cortex and how it functioned?

Deciding to test this possibility, I imagined the forward and up area of my brain and thought of shifting my attention to that area— as if aiming a light forward and up in a darkened room. Shortly afterward my eyes moved upward in their sockets, and I seemed to be more aware of both myself, and the room around me. Was I imagining it or was I also feeling strangely lighter, as if a heavy cloak had been lifted from my body?

I repeated the thought to not tighten my neck. The old, familiar response came rushing back as my attention focused downward again, as though my mind was actively searching for my neck. Then I tried my new method, saying to myself, "Think of rising forward and up to your prefrontal cortex as you think of not tightening your neck." Although I had an uneasy sense that I was not concentrating hard enough, after a few moments my breathing deepened, my back muscles released, and a subtle feeling of expansion and lightness spread through me.

Intrigued, I experimented as I sat in a chair and told myself to let my attention shift forward and up. Then I told myself to think of not standing. Soon I experienced a sense of release and ease similar to what I had noticed lying down. Feeling more confident, I decided to go ahead and stand up. Instantly my old tension came rushing back. I sat down again, repeated my thought of letting my attention rise forward and up to my prefrontal cortex and told myself to think of not standing. The tension melted away.

Then I decided to stand again, and again the muscular effort returned. This time, however, I noticed that a fraction of a second before I started to move my mind seemed to shift gears. The moment I made the decision to stand my attention shifted downward, abandoning the thought of forward and up. My mind seemed to be focused on feeling my body. As I stood up, I also noticed a silent inner dialogue: "Don't pull your knees together, that's it, now don't pull your head back; okay, remember to bend at your hips, keep your heels down; good, oops, don't hunch your shoulders." My efforts to think in this new way—shifting my attention upward as I told myself not to stand—evaporated as soon as I decided to move. Once I was in motion, my mind focused its attention on my body, trying to keep track of all my parts by feeling them, deciding what to do, and checking on what was happening.

It seemed I had reached an impasse. I could decide to stand, respond with my usual downward focus and excess muscular tension, and stand up. Or I could shift my attention forward and up, tell myself not to stand, and experience the tension falling away—but remain in the chair.

Discouraged but stubbornly refusing to quit, I decided to make things easier for myself by moving just a part of my body. I lay down on my back again, and put my left leg on the floor. I bent my right leg at the hip and knee, placing my right foot on the floor near my pelvis. I decided to notice what happened as I thought of bending my left leg, and moved it into position alongside the right.

The instant I made the decision to bend my leg, I felt an array of muscles tensing—not just in my left leg, but also in the muscles of my back, neck, and stomach. I repeated the movement

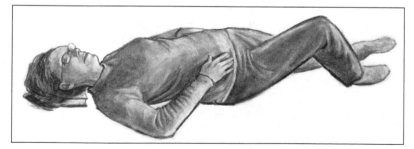

12-1. Lying in semisupine and bending the right leg. Muscles are working unnecessarily in the neck, back, abdomen, and pelvis.

many times. Every time the same pattern of muscular effort was triggered (see Illustration 12-1). Surely this effort was necessary, I told myself. A leg has weight. It requires work to move it.

But this much work?

I told myself to aim my attention upward again. This time I imagined my brain like a house with several stories, and thought of this particular area of my brain—the prefrontal cortex—as my brain's **attic**, the highest area within myself. I told myself to shift my attention upward again to my attic as I thought, over and over, "I am *not* moving my leg."* Succeeding waves of heaviness rolled off my bones as muscles that I had not even known I was tensing released their grip. But anxiety began rising within me, as if to fill the void left by the absence of my tension. I was still at the same roadblock.

How can I move my leg if I am telling myself not to move it?

Then one day I realized that I *believed* I could not move my leg because when I thought of not moving and released my muscle tension, my leg did not *feel* as if I could move it. By contrast, when I had the slightest thought to bend my leg, in an instant a familiar feeling of muscular effort arose again within me, alerting my mind that my leg was ready to move. At what seemed to be the same moment, my attention shifted downward (out of my "attic" and into my mental "basement") and then I moved. But when I thought of *not* moving, there was no answering sensation of muscular readiness. Amid the bodily silence my mind *filled in the blank*—no feeling of leg, no leg to move. I felt as if I had entered a strange never-never land, where I had been commanded to row but did not have a boat.

The next step, then, was to see if I could ignore this lack of sensation, as well as the judgment that I made about its meaning. I had to think of not moving and move my leg, without needing to *feel* as if the leg was ready to move and triggering my belief that I could move.

How do I do that?

Recalling Alexander's advice to spend lots of time inhibiting, I thought again of rising up to my attic, and repeated that I was not moving my leg. I further reminded myself that I had to make a commitment to follow through on my thought. This had to be an hon-

---

*The concept of learning to think from the attic is central to my theory of conscious inhibition. It is discussed at greater length at the end of this chapter. You will also have the opportunity to learn this skill in the self-experiments, section C.

est trial—no thinking of not moving while subtly sabotaging my effort by getting ready to move and feeling my leg. So I spent long, frustrating sessions lying on the floor with my leg straight, thinking of moving and feeling the tension rising up; then thinking up to my attic and not moving my leg; then forgetting my attic and deciding to move as I felt my tension rise up again; then erasing this effort with my inhibiting thought . . . but still not moving.

Gradually, however, I seemed to be learning something. I began paying more attention to my thought of rising forward and up to my attic. I noticed more readily when my mind shifted down into what I was more readily recognizing as my mental basement, focusing on feeling the sensations in my body as if trying to locate their source. As I continued practicing, I became better able to notice when I stopped thinking of my attic, and to resume this thought. In time I had a new ability to *know what I was thinking as I was thinking it.* This was a significant discovery—that my thought of shifting my attention forward and up to my attic, and knowing that I was thinking this thought, were not precisely the same. They were separate activities that needed to exist simultaneously. I had to both think of my attic and know I was thinking of it, as I thought of not moving.

Gradually, a new awareness of my leg seemed to emerge in my mind. It arose not so much from the feeling of my leg but from somewhere deep in my mind as I thought the word "leg." I did not have to go down to my mental basement, searching for the feeling of my leg. I could remain up in my attic, think of not moving, and *summon the meaning of the word in my mind.** With this new, broader awareness, I seemed to experience a greater sense of myself as a whole, rather than as a collection of many parts. I had a brief image of myself as a queen on her throne, waiting as her subjects (the meaning of my words) arrived to pay court.

Now I became able to frame in my mind an **intention** to move. I was able to be aware that I *wanted* to move my leg without actually *deciding* to do it. This intention was subtle, but critically different from my old way of deciding to do a movement. I knew what I *wanted* to do, but I did not decide to do it.

---

* I use this phrase to refer to the capacity of the brain to learn the meaning of words, and to transform this meaning into neurological activity that becomes embodied—that can affect us mentally, physically, and behaviorally. I am not referring to specific synonyms for a given word but to the subcortical processing of words in the brain.

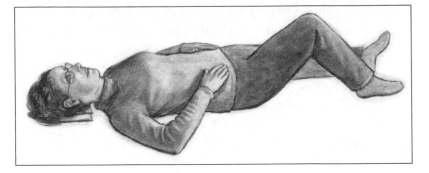

12-2. Lying in semisupine and bending the right leg while inhibiting. There is no unnecessary work in the musculature. The neck and torso are lengthened and the pelvis is not rotated.

I became so fascinated by tracking these subtle shifts in my mind's attention, awareness, meaning, and intention that my leg—and the original task of bending it—lost its urgency. Then one day, while juggling these emerging skills, suddenly, without any conscious decision or preparatory signal from my body, my leg bent and moved alongside my other leg (Illustration 12-2). More impressive was that there was not a glimmer of feeling of effort in the muscles of my neck, torso, back, or other leg as I moved. My body did nothing. This was an entirely new way of moving that seemed to require no effort. Astonishment is barely adequate to describe my reaction.

How did this happen?

Immediately I doubted myself. I must have imagined it. Summoning my courage, I tried again. Muscular tension reasserted itself as a decision to move my leg scampered across my mind. Then I used my new skills. After about five minutes, my leg bent. My muscles did not react in anticipation and overeagerness, overshooting the mark with excessive effort. I had done the movement, yet it seemed I had not *done* anything!

Over the succeeding weeks I continued practicing. Then I tried lifting an arm. Each time I found myself marveling at this new way of moving my body. I felt giddy with a happiness that is hard to describe, born not of something funny but of the ridiculous: that moving my body could prove to be so much simpler and easier than I had ever imagined; that I had spent my life hauling around these heavy limbs, when in fact they were not heavy at all!

I returned to the chair. Shifting my attention up to my attic and telling myself not to stand, once again my tension arose within me, unbidden, like an overeager hostess offering platefuls of food to her sated guests. I reminded myself not to decide to do the movement or to focus on a feeling, but to rise up to my attic and think of not standing while summoning the meaning of these words in my mind. I reminded myself of my intention to move while also thinking of not moving. After I do not know how long, I stood up. I had not decided to stand and yet I stood. It did not seem real, but the fact that I was standing was inescapable. My new way of thinking—whatever was happening neurologically—was releasing me from the grip of my habits, enabling me to move in a way that was different from anything I had ever experienced before—except that it was remarkably similar to what I had experienced in London. There was virtually nothing to feel, as some other force seemed to take charge and orchestrate my movements for me. At last I seemed to be redirecting my movements just as Alexander described, "by means of thought alone."

SURPRISES AND BELIEFS

I tried my new inhibitory skill while teaching and experienced an array of surprising benefits. I was less tired at the end of the day. Freed from my intense overfocus on feeling my body as I moved, I was able to broaden my awareness. I was no longer giving all my attention either to myself or to my student. I had a new ability to be aware of both of us, simultaneously. I was more observant. I felt more balanced emotionally. Students' problems did not bother me as much and I was less critical of myself.

I began to better appreciate the importance of Alexander's suggestion to inhibit with such broad, nonspecific instructions as "I'm not going to stand," or "I'm not going to speak." This was very different from my previous method of giving instructions to myself about a particular part of my body that needed to stop doing a particular thing. I had believed I could not inhibit successfully unless I knew which muscles were making my back tighten, for example, where they were located in my body, and the nature of their action so that I could tell myself, specifically, what they should do differently. My way of knowing this had been to focus my attention on the feelings coming from my muscles. While this *knowing-by-feeling* did help in a fashion, it only improved the mechanics of the parts of myself. It did not produce an all-encompassing effect of effortless motion throughout my whole body.

I noticed that this new way of thinking was also altering my role: I stopped worrying about whether I had changed, and whether the way that I moved was correct. I worried less in general. I began to trust that a new way of coordinating my body would emerge by itself, since it seemed governed by something other than my conscious mind. I was released from my tendency to work too hard, trying to be right.

Since my new way of thinking was having such an impact on my teaching and my use of myself, I wondered how else it might be applied. One night I was awakened from a deep sleep by a sharp spasm in my belly. Getting up to move did not help, nor did having something to eat. Returning to bed, I decided I had nothing to lose by experimenting. I thought of rising forward and up to my attic and said to myself, "I don't know what is causing this, but perhaps in some way I am doing this to myself. Whatever it is that I am doing, I want to NOT do it." After about ten minutes of repeating this thought I fell asleep. In the morning I realized with a jolt that, sometime in the middle of the night, my pain had completely disappeared.*

The next day I was lying in semisupine nervously awaiting a new student. I went up to my attic and said to myself, "I'm not teaching today." My prelesson anxiety faded away.

On another occasion I found myself unable to sleep and worrying how I would manage the next day's schedule. "I don't have anything to do tomorrow," I said to myself and drifted off to sleep.

At another time I began suffering from acid indigestion. After a week of intermittent, increasing discomfort, I decided to try inhibiting. I put myself in semisupine and went up to my attic and thought, "I don't know how I'm doing this to myself but I want to stop doing it." I repeated this for about twenty minutes but there was no improvement. I decided not to expect an immediate change, but instead to spend time each day inhibiting this reaction in myself. On the third day my symptoms disappeared and did not return.

Made miserable every spring by a sneezing, itchy nose and watery eyes, one day I noticed that when I woke in the morning my nose was clear, but a few minutes later—once I became aware

---

* I am not suggesting that conscious inhibition be a substitute for appropriate medical diagnosis and treatment; I always recommend that students with any physical complaints be examined by a physician. I am attempting to show, however, that our manner of overfocusing our mind's attention on painful sensations seems to trigger the body to overreact in a way that compounds our experience of these sensations.

of the itching sensation in my nose—it became stuffed up again. Did I have a habit of reacting to the itch, once I became aware of it, in a way that was causing my nose to become stuffed up? I went to my attic and thought, "I'm not reacting to this itch." I did this for ten minutes whenever the irritating stimulus became too great. While not disappearing entirely, gradually my allergic reactions diminished to the extent that I significantly reduced my use of antihistamines.

These experiments and others taught me that I was all too frequently reacting to an array of sensations in my body—from the feeling of my muscles tensing as I moved to other pains and discomforts large and small that arose, day and night, in an unending stream. These sensations drew my attention. The longer they lasted, the more keenly my mind tuned to them, as it focused like a beam on the area of my body from which they arose. Then I reacted in a way that perpetuated and magnified them, like sound waves reverberating against invisible inner walls. In some way, I was making these feelings stronger and the problems that arose from them worse.

During a period of high stress due to painful personal events, I practiced my inhibiting. I spent time every day lying on my back, reminding myself to go up to my attic, then telling myself not to react to the emotional pain I was experiencing. This was not repression or denial. I knew what was happening and how I felt. I understood my difficulties. I was not trying to get rid of my painful emotions but rather *not to react to them.* My tendency to overfocus on these disturbing feelings made them grow in my awareness, like watching black clouds looming on the horizon. My nervous system became overcharged, unable to rest. This was unnecessary, I told myself, and I knew how to prevent it.

I was rewarded for my practice with a greater mental clarity and calm than I had thought possible under the circumstances. I was able to sleep at night and maintain a relatively peaceful frame of mind during the day as I worked. The emotional intensity released its hold on my attention. There was a new flexibility in my mental state that allowed me to think of my problems from a different perspective. I noticed more readily when my mind reverted to its old habits, reattaching itself to sensations of pain, worry, and grief. Then I thought of inhibiting and unlocked the emotional clasp that held me. Knowing my difficulties, friends often asked, "How are you able to keep functioning?"

"It's the Alexander Technique," I answered.

Next I turned my attention to my students. Could I teach them what I had discovered? I watched them closely. As my students followed my instructions to "free the neck," or to prevent a particular physical habit such as pulling the head back, or to think of not standing, I noticed their eyes move down as their attention zoomed inward to focus on a specific part of their body. Their faces became more strained and serious. Although I was asking them to think of not doing anything, instead they were trying to feel, deciding what should change in their body, and doing something muscularly to try to change it.

One day I asked a student to imagine his attention shifting "forward and up" within himself, as if turning on a light in the area of his mind above his eyes. It seemed a long shot, but I noticed his downward gaze shift up and out, and I felt tension release from his musculature. Encouraged, I tried again on my next student. This student had come to me complaining of severe neck tension. In the early lessons I could barely turn her head. Over several months this had improved only slightly. Then I taught her to rise up to her attic and think of not tightening her neck. I was able to turn her head with ease in a matter of seconds.

Since then many other students have had similar, sudden releases of tension. Others have become lighter and easier to move. People with chronic pain have reported significant lessening of their pain. Still others have described themselves feeling calmer, less depressed, and sleeping better. A richer world of exploration has opened to them as they have learned to inhibit consciously and skillfully.

Along with my success with this approach, however, I have encountered an unexpected challenge—the problem of belief. Few students believe me when I tell them that how they think can become a vital tool for reducing stress, remedying pain and injury, and enhancing their lives. Since they do not believe me, they do not fully engage in the process of learning to inhibit and so do not experience the same results. Then they fail to discover that it is their belief that keeps them from experiencing inhibition's rewards.

A fascinating experiment published in the *American Journal of Psychiatry* studied patients with depression. Half were given antidepressants, the other half a placebo. About the same number of patients in each group reported improvement in their symptoms. But follow-up brain scans gave a different picture. Those on placebo showed increased activity in their prefrontal cortex. Those taking the antidepressants did not; their scans appeared the same as before taking the medication.[11]

This study lends support to theories about the role of the prefrontal cortex in regulating mood. But it has another important message. People who experience improvement in any of a variety of symptoms after taking a sugar pill have long been derided as victims of a self-induced hoax. It now appears that such people are succeeding where most of us cannot. Through their belief that they are on medication, they are rerouting their brain's activity in healthful ways. They are not consciously deciding to do this. They have no awareness it is happening. What is the active agent? Their belief that they are taking a medication that will cure their problem. By taking a pill, even a sugar pill, they are thinking differently; they are thinking of overcoming their symptoms. In turn, their mind appears to figure out how to realize this thought.*

In an interesting epilogue to this study, when those on placebo who experienced improvement in their depression were told they had been on a placebo, their symptoms returned—all except for one individual, who correctly concluded that taking the pill caused him to think differently, which enabled him to overcome his depression. He sustained his improvement.

This study helps us understand how it may be that a mere belief can affect our health. The obstacle is not always in our genes, physiology, or in some noxious outside agent. It may be in our manner of thinking. The catch-22 in teaching students to inhibit is that, in order for them to experience its effectiveness they must believe that it can be effective, but often they are not willing to believe it can be effective until they have experienced its effectiveness. I suggest that they try suspending their disbelief and behave *as if* it were true. Afterward, I assure them, they can readily return to disbelieving.

If this does not shift their unyielding doubt I try another experiment. I ask my student to make a fist. As her fingers curl around her palm, I pose a question. "How did you do that?" My student does not reply. She has never considered the question.

---

* I am not suggesting that we can cure all illness simply by thinking. I am attempting to show that recent research is shedding new light on the connection between mind and body, and the increasing evidence for the mind's capacity to hinder or enhance our health.

"Of course, we don't have the whole answer to this, but we can say that at some point in your life you learned to understand the meaning of each of the words "Make a fist." You didn't understand their meaning when you were an infant. Then you learned to say the words to yourself in a precise way that decoded their meaning into neural signals that made the right connections to the right muscles so that your fingers bent when you asked them to. Your thought makes that happen. If you can learn to think to *do* something—to make a fist—you can learn to think *not* to do something. You can think, *I'm* not *making a fist*. The thought of doing excites neurons to produce a muscular response. The thought of not doing can *lessen the excitation of neurons to prevent a response*. This is conscious inhibition. It is as important a capacity of the nervous system as excitation. In fact, it is more important.

"Why is it so important?" I ask. "Stimuli are coming at you all the time, day and night, via all your sensory systems: eyes, ears, nose, bodily sensations, even your thoughts. These stimuli trigger nerves to fire. Once nerves are firing they also stimulate neurons to double back and restimulate the initial neuron in a self-regenerating loop. Our sensory systems act like a perpetual 'go' message. When we experience too much input, we become stressed. Our nerves can't stop firing. Our amygdala keeps working. We can't relax and unwind. We can't turn off.

"In addition, your every movement requires that some muscles work, while others do not work (inhibition). When you cannot let go of your muscles at the appropriate moment as you move, your coordination is impeded. Then you only work harder in an effort to counter this self-induced resistance.

"Conscious inhibition is the cheapest, safest, and simplest method available to countermand your nervous system's overactivity. It is the crucial first step to achieve a more skilled use of your body in motion. You don't have to numb yourself with alcohol, take sleeping pills or drugs. You don't have to go on vacation. You don't have to spend long periods of time stretching muscles. You can consciously tell yourself to bring your attention forward and up to your attic to deactivate the tension and stress within you. It's free. It's available anytime, anywhere. You have only to believe it is possible and practice it."

IT HAS BEEN a long journey since the day I stood in Carrington's teaching room enjoying my lesson and a fine summer afternoon in London. I had no idea then what was in store for me. Looking back, I see that I was perched on the crest of a wave, soon to be swept along by an experience I did not understand but could not ignore. It is no exaggeration to say this lesson changed my life. Since then, I have learned how to recognize the difference between rising up to my attic to think of inhibiting, and going down to my mental basement to focus on feeling. I can distinguish between deciding to do an action versus framing an intention to move in my mind. I can generate a fuller awareness of the whole of myself as I summon the meaning of words in my mind. And I have a new understanding of the role of belief in determining behavior. Our beliefs are not abstract ideas that we form, separate and apart from our physical self. They arise from the mind's interpretation and extrapolation of sensory experience. Through inhibition I have learned to move more skillfully, and as a result I have become better able to change my beliefs.

In the next chapter we will see how belief gets in my son's way as he tries to hit a baseball, and how conscious inhibition helps him bat with startling success.

13

Believing Is Not Seeing

Ninety-nine percent of the game is half mental.
—YOGI BERRA

WHEN MY SON, Jared, was nine years old he joined the Little League. It was not long into the season before he came home from practice one day crying in frustration.

"What's wrong?" I asked.

"I struck out every time at bat."

"Let's go to the field tomorrow after school. I'll throw and watch you hit. Maybe I can help," I offered.

"What do you know about batting?" he challenged.

"You might be surprised," I said, hoping to keep the conversation open.

Jared responded with a roll of his eyes and a smirk, letting me know how doubtful he was about his mother being of any use to him in this department, but he nodded his head and silently agreed to give me a try.

On the field the next day, Jared stood in position by the plate as I stood on the mound. I threw the ball and watched in dismay. Jared's neck muscles tensed, pulling his head back and down into his neck. His shoulders squeezed together and his hands gripped the bat. His knees pressed together as his leg muscles clenched and his body crouched toward the ground. By the time the ball reached the plate he was a study in tension. Channeling all his energy into his arms, he swung his bat with furious intensity and missed the ball completely.

Feeling a mixture of concern and relief, I knew I didn't have to be Babe Ruth or Sherlock Holmes to discern the source of his problem.

"Jared," I said, "you need to keep your eyes on the ball."

"I am!" he threw back at me.

"No, you really aren't watching the ball," I repeated.

"I am, too!" he insisted, his voice rising.

How to help? Telling Jared that he was not keeping his eyes on the ball was not going to do it. He firmly believed this was exactly what he was doing. Disagreeing with him was not going to change his belief. Shifting my approach, I asked what advice his coach had given him.

"Swing hard and hit a home run," he answered.

These were end-gaining instructions if ever there were any. Jared was entirely absorbed in thinking about his goal of hitting a home run and had no patience for thinking about the best way to do it. I had to find a way to get him out of his goal-oriented mind-set and to open his mind to the idea that he needed to learn to watch the ball. I knew if he did not give up trying so hard to hit a home run, he would never get to first base. But how to explain inhibiting to a nine-year-old, convince him not to think about hitting home runs, and to relinquish his belief long enough to teach him to see the ball?

"Jared, let's do this some more. I'll throw and you hit. Let's see what happens."

Jared stood at the plate, arms up, bat high over his shoulder. He looked pretty good. As soon as I began to throw, however, his body changed. All the malcoordinating tension came rushing back. The ball was a stimulus to which he reacted in an instant, triggering his belief that he had to swing hard to hit a home run. Was there a way to trick him into thinking differently, just long enough to give him a new experience of batting? If I could do that much he might begin to shift his belief and learn to see the ball. I decided to try something radical.

"Jared," I said, "Let's try something different. It's very simple. Stand at the plate and hold the bat the way you usually do. I'm going to throw the ball, but I don't want you to move your bat. Leave it where it is. Tell yourself not to swing. All I want you to do is watch the ball as it moves toward you. Keep watching the ball as it approaches you, as it crosses the plate, and even as it passes by you. See it the entire time it's moving. You don't have to do anything else. Got it?"

"Okay," he answered. In a single word Jared's voice expressed a mound of doubt. I ignored him and pitched. After the ball passed by him, I asked if he'd seen it the entire time that it was in the air.

"I think so," he answered.

"Let's try it again."

I pitched. "What about this time? Did you see the ball the entire time it was moving?"

"That's weird."

"What's weird?"

"I saw the ball as it was coming toward me, but when it was about three feet in front of me it sort of disappeared. Then I saw it again after it passed by me. That's really weird. How'd that happen?"

While Jared was feeling puzzled, I was feeling hopeful. If he could perceive that he had stopped seeing the ball, we had something I could work with—an experience that might cause him to change his belief.

"That's great. You're starting to know what it means to see the ball. You have to see it clearly during the entire time that it's traveling toward you. When it sort of disappears like that, it means you've stopped seeing it. When you tell me you're not sure if you saw the ball that means you didn't really see it. Want to try this again?"

Jared nodded. He stood in position, engaged now in the challenge of watching the ball and noticing when it mysteriously disappeared from view. I threw the ball and watched carefully. Even from my pitcher's distance it was clear, from the movement of his head, when he stopped seeing the ball. When he was seeing it, his head turned smoothly and evenly. When he lost sight of it, his head stopped for just a split second, making the overall movement appear less smooth.

"I stopped seeing it again, Mom," Jared announced. "I lost it again. This time I lost it just as the ball was almost in front of me."

"That's great. You're learning to see the ball and you're learning to recognize when you've stopped seeing it. This is what you want to practice. It doesn't happen automatically, you have to learn it. Let's keep doing this for a while."

I threw. Jared watched. I threw some more. Jared kept watching. His concentration had shifted and he was focused keenly on seeing the ball. With each pitch he reported more success at seeing the ball the entire time that it moved toward him. After about fifteen minutes he was consistently seeing the ball through its entire arc of travel. More important, he knew when he'd stopped seeing it—even for just a split second—and was often able to find it again.

In this short period Jared had changed into an eager student. By removing the act of swinging his bat and the accompanying frustration of not being able to hit, he could put his mind on his task. The activity was teaching him, as no amount of arguing possibly could, that he had not been doing what he believed he was doing. After a while he was reporting consistent success.

"What's next?" he asked with enthusiasm. My son was eagerly awaiting my next instruction, while I tried to figure out what that was. What could be an intermediate step between not swinging the bat and swinging it hard to hit a home run?

"Okay," I said after some thought, "here's the next step. This time keep watching the ball. Then let your bat move until the ball is right in front of you, but don't follow through with your swing. I want you to stop your swing when the ball is right in front of you. If you keep your mind on watching the ball, then you should see the ball and the bat make contact. See the ball and the bat touch, but don't swing the bat any farther. Got it?"

"Okay."

Jared stood in batting position as I threw. I watched as the old tension rose again in his body. It seemed he could not help himself. With permission to move his bat, Jared's old thinking returned—swing hard. He tensed himself in his usual way, did not stop the bat as I had instructed, and definitely did not keep his eyes on the ball. He missed it completely. But he looked up at me immediately afterward and said, "I didn't keep my eyes on the ball, Mom. I lost it."

"That's great, Jared. You knew that you stopped seeing it. What were you thinking about, could you tell?"

"I was thinking about hitting a home run."

"Aha! So while you were thinking about hitting a home run, what weren't you thinking?"

"I didn't keep thinking about seeing the ball."

"You've got it. Then your body did just what you told it to do. You thought about trying to hit a home run, so your body became tense. Since you were thinking about hitting hard, you stopped thinking about seeing. I know it's difficult to believe, but if you can stop thinking about trying to hit a home run and put your mind instead on seeing the ball, the chances are much better that you'll actually hit a home run. Let's go back to the first step and practice watching the ball without moving the bat."

I pitched as Jared held his bat over his shoulder and watched. We practiced until he was seeing the ball throughout its entire arc of travel. Then we moved on to the next step of seeing the bat make contact with the ball in front of him. Again Jared met with failure. After several more misses he threw his bat on the ground in frustration and sat down in the dirt.

"Jared, what were you thinking about?"

"I was thinking about when to swing my bat so I could see it touch the ball like you asked," he answered, exasperated.

"But that's not what I asked you to do."

"What do you mean?"

"I didn't ask you to think about swinging your bat, I asked you to think about watching the ball and then to allow your bat to move to meet it."

"What's the difference?"

"That's a good question. It's a crucial difference. When I threw the ball, you shifted your thinking and focused your mind on your arms and deciding when to swing. But when you did that, you forgot to keep seeing the ball."

"If I'm not supposed to focus on my arms and think about swinging my bat, how am I going to know when to swing?" he demanded. "I have to decide to swing my bat!" Jared's voice was rising. I left the mound and walked over to him. In as calm a voice as I could muster I said, "Jared, I know you don't believe me yet, but the swing will do itself. Really it will. Remember the first step, when I told you not to swing your bat and all you had to do was keep watching the ball?"

"Yeah."

"Since you didn't have to swing the bat, you didn't think about it, right?"

"Yeah."

"That's what you want to keep doing even when you swing your bat. When you think about your bat, you change how you're thinking about seeing the ball. Instead, you want to allow your arms to move the bat without paying so much attention to them. You've learned to really focus your mind on feeling your muscles working as you move, and feeling your arms swinging your bat. But that distracts you from what you want to be thinking. You want to learn to keep your mind on watching the ball." As I spoke, I could not ignore Jared's skeptical expression.

"I know this sounds pretty strange," I added.

"You bet it does."

"Jared, just try it. What have you got to lose? Prove me wrong. But prove me wrong by trying it, okay?"

"I can't believe what you're telling me, Mom. You want me to tell myself not to swing the bat, but you want me to swing the bat and let it touch the ball? That's ridiculous."

"Think of it as magic. If you make up your mind to keep watching the ball, another part of your brain will take in the information about the ball's speed and direction, process it, and figure out the right moment to swing. You don't have to do that. In a sense you have a **helper** inside of you, who will know the right moment to move your arms and swing for you. When you decide to swing by focusing on feeling your arms, you're getting in the way of your helper. And you quit doing what you want to be doing, which is keeping your mind on seeing the ball. You can't possibly figure out the right moment to move your bat. Your conscious mind can't do that. It doesn't know the right moment to swing. But if you keep your mind on watching the ball, the information will be processed in your brain and another part of your mind will do the swing for you. Trust me. Let's try it again. You'll see what I mean in a minute."

Jared did not answer but he stood up, walked to get his bat, and then stood in position as I walked to the pitcher's mound.

"Tell yourself not to swing, Jared. You don't have to worry about the swing. Your helper will do it for you. Just keep seeing the ball."

I pitched. As I watched it was clear Jared was keeping his mind on the ball. His head turned easily, poised freely on his neck. His shoulders didn't hunch and his legs didn't clutch. As the ball neared the plate, his arms began smoothly into motion. There were none of the previous mannerisms of tensing to get ready to hit. He simply stood, watching the ball, while his arms began moving the bat in a smooth arc. Then the bat and ball made contact in front of him. Jared stopped the bat's forward movement just as I instructed. His timing was perfect.

"I saw it! I actually saw the bat touch the ball, Mom!" he exclaimed.

I felt relieved but aloud I said, "That's what I'm talking about, Jared. You don't have to think about your arms and decide to swing your bat. Let your helper do that for you. Your job is to tell yourself not to swing. And to think of seeing the ball."

We practiced for ten minutes. Occasionally Jared would revert to tensing and trying to swing too hard. Each time he did, he looked up at me afterward and said, "I was thinking about swinging my arms again, Mom. I didn't keep thinking about seeing the ball."

Gradually the activity was making my case for me. Jared was learning to recognize when he reverted to thinking about hitting a home run and deciding to swing his bat. Each time, this caused him to react by getting tense and losing sight of the ball. Among other things, the experience was a powerful lesson for my son in the pitfalls of end-gaining.

"Okay. Now you're seeing the ball and coordinating this with the movement of your arms," I said. "Let's add one more step. This time you can let your bat keep moving. Keep thinking about not swinging and just seeing the ball, but allow your bat to keep moving. Don't stop the swing. Got it?"

"Yeah."

I pitched again. Jared missed. With the new instruction, again he stopped focusing his attention on seeing the ball.

"I didn't see the ball," he quickly confessed, "I didn't keep thinking what you told me to think." We reviewed the first two steps. When he was back on track, we went on to the swing. I pitched and watched as Jared focused, kept his eyes on the ball, and followed its movement. His mind was focused on seeing. Then his arms began to move, his bat traveling smoothly and easily in its arc. There was no undue strain or tension in his body. The ball and bat connected as Jared's arms continued moving. It was a straight, clean drive past me to second base.

"Wow!" Jared said in astonishment. "I wasn't even trying to hit it!"

"That was great, Jared!"

"That's cool!" By now Jared's resistance had vanished. He was absorbed in the learning process and proud of his accomplishment. We continued practicing. My pitches were erratic—too low, too high, outside, inside. Jared kept seeing the ball and making contact. He almost never missed and the majority of his hits were straight drives past me, which indicated not only a new accuracy in seeing the ball but a consistency in timing his swing. Finally we went home to dinner.

As I was saying good night later that evening Jared said, "You know what was really amazing about this batting stuff we did today, Mom?"

"What?"

"When it worked, I really wasn't thinking about my bat, or swinging my arms, or trying to hit the ball. I didn't decide to swing my bat. I just thought about seeing the ball like you told me, and my arms moved at the right time. I didn't have to think about my arms or the bat. It was like I didn't have to do anything!"

A smile spread across my face as I answered, "That's what I teach people—to think of not doing, while letting their helper do the work for them."

"You know a lot about baseball, Mom."

There was a wondering smile on Jared's face and, I am sure, no small expression of pride on my own. My son was quietly expressing his respect and admiration for what his mom, a mere girl, had been able to teach him about baseball. (Yet another citadel of belief was dashed on that day.)

Other than occasionally thinking with pleasure about the remainder of Jared's Little League career that season, during which he failed only once to have a hit at bat, I did not give our experiment any further thought. Several years later, however, students enrolled in my teacher-training course asked to apply the Technique to sports. I decided to try the batting experiment with them. I am not sure what I was expecting, but I was not expecting it to be the success that it was with Jared. I was wrong. With each student, the problems and tensions were virtually the same. They could not keep watching the ball when they swung the bat. Later, when they mastered seeing the ball and were told to move their bats, they lost their visual coordination again as they focused on feeling their arms and deciding to swing.

After they learned to see the ball and think of not swinging in order to let their helper move the bat as they simply watched the bat and ball make contact, I asked them to follow through with the swing. Invariably they stopped seeing the ball again. When they finally managed all three steps, their comments were remarkably the same.

"Wow! I didn't swing the bat. It swung itself."

"I didn't have to decide to do it! That's amazing!"

"How'd that happen?"

It was not until years later that a student offered to pitch and let me have a chance to try my own experiment. Afflicted with poor vision and bad depth perception from an early age, I had long since given up on ball sports. I picked up the bat and faced my pitcher with trepidation. Fifteen minutes later, just like those before me, my bat found the ball. There was a satisfying thwack as the ball flew forward.

"Amazing!" I heard myself saying. "I didn't swing the bat!"

14

The Difference That Inhibition Makes

Human beings, by changing the inner attitudes of their minds,
can change the outer aspects of their lives.

—WILLIAM JAMES

ERIN, PART TWO

WE MET ERIN in chapter 2 as she was introduced to the Technique. Since then she has had about six weekly lessons. Today she is standing in front of the chair in my teaching room. We are beginning what teachers call a "chair lesson." The purpose of this is not so much to teach the right way to sit and stand as it is to give the student an opportunity to observe and become aware of his or her malcoordinating patterns of movement, and to practice inhibiting as the teacher moves him or her in and out of the chair. The student must also sustain this thinking in the midst of the powerful stimulus of being moved by the teacher. The chair lesson presents a particular challenge, since students must also deal with gravity and the instinctive fear of falling.

"Okay, Erin, I'm going to support you and help you to sit. I'll do much of the work. I have my hand on your back so you can't fall. As I do this, I'd like you to inhibit. Think to yourself, 'I'm not sitting down.'"

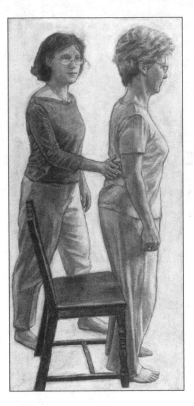

14-1. Erin standing habitually with her neck stiffened back, head forward and down, shoulders and arms pulled back, fingers curled, and lower back arched.

Erin nods her head. I begin by moving her back slightly from her ankles to shift her weight over her heels as I support her with my hand on her back. If she does not tense unnecessarily, this will help her legs to release forward to counterbalance the backward movement of her torso. This, in turn, will help her to sit.

As I move Erin back, however, my hands feel an almost instantaneous reaction. The muscles in her neck and upper back shorten and become hard. Her body feels heavier in my hand. Her lower back arches as she readies herself to sit. In the next instant her thigh muscles tense as well and her legs become stiffer. I move Erin's body forward to return her to the vertical standing position (Illustration 14-1).

"Erin, what did you notice just then? I moved you back just a little bit. Can you say what happened to your thinking? Did you keep thinking about not sitting down?"

Erin hesitates. "Well, sort of . . . now that you mention it, I guess I was thinking about sitting in the chair."

"Were you inhibiting?"

"No, I guess not."

"Did you notice what happened as I moved you?"

"I think I got more tense in my back."

"Right. Do you need to do that?"

"Well, don't I have to do some work to sit down?"

"If you were going to sit down by yourself, of course you would. But we agreed that I would support you and move you, while you think of not sitting so that you don't tense your muscles. If we work together in this way, you will have an experience of sitting that will be coordinated differently than the way you usually do it.

"In order to begin, I'm taking you slightly back on your ankles as I support you. All you have to do is think of not sitting. Let's try it again. Remember that you don't have to sit yourself down. Let me move you."

I repeat the same procedure but as soon as I begin, I feel the same reaction in Erin's body. Without speaking I move her to the vertical and try again. The same thing happens. I move her to the vertical again.

"Erin, what did you notice as I moved you?"

Erin looks chagrined. "I can't get my muscles to stop tightening."

"That isn't what I'm asking of you."

"What do you mean?"

"I'm asking you to inhibit. That's just a thought. You can't do anything, directly, to keep your muscles from tightening. If you try, you'll only tense them more."

"How am I going to sit down?"

"Let's think about this. We've seen that you react as I move you by overtensing your back muscles, right?"

"Yeah."

"This is your habit. It's what you do every time you sit—you tense your back muscles too much."

"Okay . . ." she answers, her voice trailing off.

"Since this is your habit, you do this every time you sit down. It's the only way you know to sit. You can't expect yourself to sit differently, because you don't know what that is or how to do it." Erin looks relieved. "I guess I don't."

"That means you're off the hook. You don't have to be a good student and get this right. It's not your job to figure out what is right, and then do the movement the right way. It's your job to *think*. You're learning to inhibit—to think of not sitting. If you do that, I'll do the rest. I'll move you in a way that will teach you about another way to use your muscles as you sit. I can't tell you how to do this. No amount of verbal instruction will give you the experience of using your muscles differently. To learn it, you have to experience it. My hands can't make your muscles let go, but they can support you and move you in a new way. If you inhibit, my hands can give you a new experience."

"Okay," Erin replies. "Let's try again."

"First, let me add that this is what everyone goes through as they begin lessons. We all have ways of moving that are inefficient and unconscious. Since we are not aware of them, we can't change them. This is what you're learning how to do in these lessons."

Erin nods. I place my right hand on her back and put my other hand on the front of her hip. I move her slightly back. Again she reacts in her habitual way.

"What happened this time?" I ask as I move her to standing.

"It's kind of scary, you know? I feel like I'm going to fall down."

"That's your brain's interpretation of the new sensations you experience as I move you, even just this small amount. I only asked you to think of inhibiting, but your mind became distracted by these feelings and then formed a judgment of their meaning. Since your brain concluded that you are falling, it also triggered a fear reaction. In the midst of all this, you stopped thinking.

"But remember, I have my hands on you. You can't fall. Remind yourself that you're not going to fall because I'm supporting you."

Erin nods her head without speaking.

"Now remind yourself you're not falling, no matter how it feels, and tell yourself not to—"

"But I just don't see how this is possible," Erin interrupts, turning to face me.

"Because?"

"I have to do work to sit down, otherwise I'd fall in a heap on the floor!" Erin says, her voice rising.

"Yes, you're right. You do have to do some work in your muscles to be upright, but the work is minimal. It's so slight that you shouldn't really feel your muscles at all. I'm only asking you to think of not sitting. I'm not asking you to completely relax."

"But I can't let you sit me down," Erin persists, as if she hasn't heard what I've said.

"Why not?"

"I feel as though I'm going to hurt you. I'm heavy. I'll knock you over."

Erin is expressing a belief, which again is based on a judgment about what she is feeling. It is also another fear. Implicit in her worry that she will make me fall down is the worry that she will fall down. By moving her just this small amount, sensations have been triggered to which her amygdala has reacted in an instant. Now she is in a freeze behavior. Her muscles have tensed even more. This makes her task of inhibiting, and my task of moving her, more difficult.

Hoping to allay her fear I say, "Erin, I've been doing this for years. I haven't dropped a student yet and no one has knocked me down either."

"I find that hard to believe."

"I understand, most people do. But that it's hard for you to believe doesn't mean you're correct. Here we are, doing just the smallest movement, and look at how many beliefs we've uncovered that you have about this one movement—beliefs that affect your behavior, your decisions, and your muscular activity. Can you suspend these beliefs for a moment? Can you behave as if they aren't correct, and simply tell yourself not to sit?"

Erin nods her head and we begin as before. This time, as I move her, her back and neck muscles do not tense; her head remains forward and up, counterbalancing her body. Since her back muscles have not tensed, her spine has not compressed.

"That's good, Erin. You're inhibiting. You're moving differently. Let me continue supporting you as you continue thinking of not sitting. You don't have to help me or try to do anything."

As I support her weight, I feel Erin's back muscles lengthening. Her chest is easing upward very slightly, lengthening away from her pelvis. She feels lighter in my hands. Next there is a release of excess tension in her abdomen and legs. Her ribs move more freely and she is breathing better. I continue to support her as her torso lengthens slightly more upward. Her leg muscles continue to release. They are no longer clutching, holding her in a habitual lock. Her legs begin

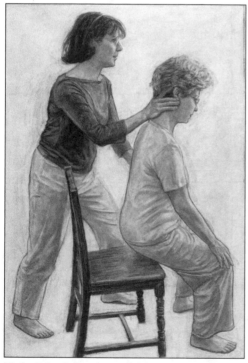

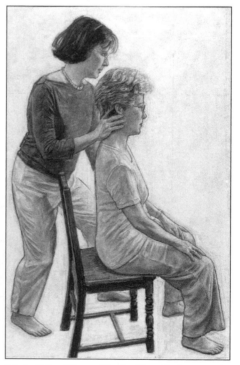

14-2. Erin sitting down with hands-on guidance from the teacher. Her neck is lengthening upward and her head is forward and up on the neck; her torso is lengthening headward and her shoulders are widening apart as her arms hang freely. Her hips, knees, and ankles are bending easily.

14-3. Erin sitting with significantly improved locomotor skill.

to bend, folding at the knees, hips, and ankles. I continue to support her as I bend as well, lowering her toward the chair (see Illustration 14-2).

A moment later, Erin is sitting in the chair (see Illustration 14-3).

"That was great, Erin. You sat down but you didn't overtense in your muscles. You inhibited your habitual way of moving by thinking of not sitting—and not focusing on your feelings and making judgments about them. You prevented your reaction. Did you notice any difference from the way you usually sit?"

"I was barely aware that I was moving. I just kept thinking of not sitting like you asked. It seemed as though I floated into the chair." She pauses. "How'd that happen?"

"You did float into the chair. You were practically weightless. This is what I mean about a new way of sitting. And you didn't relax entirely, or you'd have landed heavily."

"How'd that happen?" she repeats.

"Well, we could say that you have a helper."

Erin smiles and looks at me.

"No, I don't mean me. Your helper is within you. When you inhibited by thinking of not sitting, another part of your brain switched into gear and adjusted the tension in your muscles so that they worked just as much as necessary—not too much, and not too little. By inhibiting you're removing the muscular interference that springs into action when your brain feels what is happening in your body and imposes its learned idea about how much effort is required. If you can stop doing that by inhibiting, other mechanisms in your brain will play a bigger role, helping to coordinate your torso upward as you bend your legs to move. I can't teach you this by telling you about it. We have to work together—your inhibiting, and my hands and verbal instruction—so you can learn to allow your helper to move you more efficiently.

"As you're seated now, do you notice anything?"

Erin turns her head to look in the mirror. "I don't believe it," she says.

"What?"

"I was going to say that you have put me in the wrong place—that you've got me leaning over, sort of slumped."

"Is that how you look in the mirror?"

"No. I look like I'm sitting up. It looks good. This sure doesn't feel like the way I usually sit. I was just about to ask why you wanted me to sit leaning forward!"

"You didn't believe you were sitting upright?"

"No, I thought I was kind of hunched forward."

"You have yet another belief based on a feeling. This time it's a belief about how it should feel when you sit."

"I guess so."

"If the mirror hadn't been here to give you this proof, what would you have done?"

Erin tenses her back muscles again, pulling her upper body backward, stiffening her neck and arching her lower back (Illustration 14-4).

"This feels right to you? This is what you believe is sitting up straight?" I ask.

"Yeah, this is what I try to do when I'm sitting. This isn't straight?" she asks.

"Look in the mirror. Take time to observe yourself. What do you see?"

Erin looks but doesn't speak.

"Imagine a plumb line dropping to the ground from the middle of your ear. Does it fall through the center of your body and down through the center of your pelvis?" I ask.

"It looks like my ear is behind my pelvis."

"What does that tell you?"

"I'm leaning back!"

"If this is how you usually sit, what is this doing to your vertebrae and disks?"

"Compressing them?"

"Right."

I use my hands to gently guide Erin to restore the balancing, upwardly lengthening torso she had a moment before.

"But I can't sit like this!" she protests.

"Because?"

"This just doesn't feel right. I can't believe this is right."

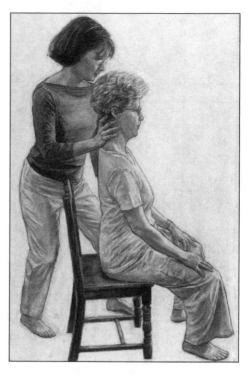

14-4. Erin reverting to her habitual pattern of tension. Her neck is stiffened and flattened, the jaw is pulled back, the upper back is overly flattened, the pelvis is tipped forward, and the lower back is arched.

"But what does the mirror tell you? Don't take my word for it. Look at yourself again." Erin's expression is still skeptical.

"Why does this seem so wrong?" she asks, her voice lower.

"This is what we call your psychophysical habit. Every time you decide to sit, you overtense your back and leg muscles, creating the feelings that your brain has learned to connect with the meaning of the word 'sit.' But all that excess tension makes it harder to bend your legs, so you become even tenser in your back muscles, trying to pull yourself down into the chair. Once you've done all that tensing in your back and legs as you sit, you land heavily in the chair. Then you hold on to all that tension as you're sitting. You never let it go. You've done this for so long it has become a habit, and that means it feels right to you. But this isn't just a habit of tensing your muscles. It's paired with your belief—it is based on a wrong interpretation of what you're feeling—that is, that you're sitting up straight when you aren't.

"Have you been told that sitting up straight is the right way to sit to help your back?"

Erin nods.

"Here you are trying to do what you believe is good for your back, but you don't know what that is or how to do it. It's true that you don't want to slump, which is bad for your disks and vertebrae. But that's not what you're doing. You haven't been sitting 'right.' You've been sitting in the way that 'feels right.'

"And now this new, better way of sitting feels wrong so you're not likely to do it, are you?"

"No!"

"You're also not likely to get rid of your back pain. Not until you learn to inhibit these habits: overtensing your muscles in everything you do, not only injuring yourself physically but also reinforcing your incorrect beliefs. I think now you can better appreciate what I mean when I say that you have an unconscious way of moving that is contributing to your back pain. And this physical tension is literally held in place by your wrong belief—that the right way to sit is the way that feels right."

You Have a Helper

*The universe is full of magical things patiently
waiting for our wits to grow sharper.*
—Eden Phillpots

S OMETIMES WE BELIEVE our body is doing what it is
not. Other times we believe our body is not doing what it is
doing. In both cases, we are misjudging bodily sensations. These
usually unconscious misperceptions prevent us from achieving
self-mastery. The advice Jared's coach gave him—to swing hard
and hit a home run and to just try harder—is typical. Unfortunately, this advice only works if you are already doing everything
right. If you are starting from a point of mind-body disconnection—unconsciously misusing your body and misjudging the
meaning of bodily feedback—trying harder only makes the
problem worse.

Common strategies for dealing with the problem of not being
able to make our body do what we want it to do include: 1) *Exercising specific muscles to increase muscle strength* in the belief that, if
something is not working right, our muscles must be weak. 2)
Stretching specific muscles to relax them in the belief that, if something is not working right, our muscles must be tight. 3) *Moving
specific parts of the body in specific ways* in the belief that we can reliably know what is wrong and what is right through feeling.

None of these approaches addresses the central problem I have been describing—that our subconscious, psychophysical habits of misuse create a distorted self-perception in the mind. Only a psychophysical approach that begins by correcting our misuse through conscious inhibition can get to the heart of the problem. In this way Jared's batting problem was solved in a short period of time. He did not need to do muscle strengthening exercises or stretches. I did not give him verbal instruction in how to hold his bat the right way and swing correctly. I did not ask him to rely on judging his feelings in order to know if he was moving correctly. Instead, I asked him to think of not swinging his bat as he practiced watching the ball. Then I asked him to think of not swinging his bat while letting his bat meet the ball. This presented a unique challenge. It is one thing to think of not doing something while you aren't doing it. It is another matter entirely to think of not doing something while you are doing it.

"Why should I do that? Isn't that impossible? How can I move when I'm thinking of *not* moving?" my students ask. I faced a similar challenge when I tried to bend my leg without deciding to bend it. Erin faced this problem when I asked her to think of not sitting while allowing me to move her. Bruce reacted negatively when I asked him to play while thinking of not playing. Inhibiting is not difficult. But when students are asked to think of not doing the activity that they are actually doing, they invariably resist. This instruction flies in the face of their belief.

In response to my students' queries and puzzled expressions I often reply, "It sounds illogical, but try it anyway. If you can suspend your disbelief and sustain your decision to think of not doing the action, magic will happen."

How does thinking of not moving enable us to move more skillfully? The answer lies in the fact that there is a great deal more to your brain than your conscious awareness. The human brain has evolved over many millions of years. As a result, we might say that we do not have one brain but several. (These are commonly referred to as the hindbrain and the midbrain—or sometimes as the "reptilian" brain—and forebrain, or the "mammalian" brain.) Another way to think of this is that as the human brain evolved, it acquired additional *operating systems*, or increasingly complex mechanisms of organization and control.

Through this process of evolution and increasing complexity, there has also been a certain replication of functions. For example, when you are asleep, the oldest part of your brain coordinates your breathing for you. (This is the original brain dating from about five hundred million years ago.) But thanks to your forebrain—the newest addition—you can become aware that it is you that breathes. You can tell yourself to override the old system of control and make yourself breathe, or allow yourself not to breathe for a time. You can also modify how you breathe by deciding to exaggerate the downward contraction of your diaphragm, or alter the movement of your ribs, or change the rate of your exhalation.

When you consciously *decide* to do a movement, or when you do a movement that you have already learned how to do, output signals are sent from your newest operating system—your forebrain—down to your body along a specific neural pathway known as the *corticospinal pathway*. This is like the front staircase in the house that is your brain. By contrast, when you use older, subcortical parts of your brain to send instructions to your body, such as breathing via your hindbrain, signals are being routed through a different neural pathway, the *extrapyramidal pathway*. This is like the back staircase in your house.

In short, your capacity to move your body derives from several overlapping brain systems. Because of the somatosensory cortex in your forebrain and the corticospinal pathway, you can consciously decide you want to make a fist, learn to move your fingers in a certain way to play the piano, or hold a racket and hit a tennis ball. This area of your brain is what enables you to learn the discrete skills involved in doing much of what you do with your body. Movement happens in large part because, once you have learned how to do it, you decide to do it.

Before the forebrain evolved, the older brain in conjunction with the cerebellum and the extrapyramidal pathway, managed the animal's locomotion quite well. (I have referred previously to these subcortical areas, acting in combination, as your "helper.") In fact, our capacity for skilled and coordinated movement evolved long before we acquired a conscious, decision-making self. How does a centipede manage to move its one hundred legs without tripping? It does not have to decide which foot to move first and when, or even learn how to walk. Its tiny nervous system handles its movements expertly. Thus, our capacity for movement happens in conjunction with older, subcortical areas of the brain. I speak of this as your helper because it plays a vital role in how you move. It is this older area, and in particular the cerebellum, that helps Michael Jordan be—well, Michael Jordan.

This is a critical difference: Because of the somatosensory cortex we can learn specific movement skills. We can learn to dribble a ball and decide to aim for the basket. Without the full assistance of our helper, however, this will be but a series of relatively disjointed and poorly coordinated acts. The conscious mind does not know how to gauge the exact amount of tension in each of our muscles at every moment appropriate to a given activity, such that each muscle works just as much as required, no more and no less. Our conscious mind does not know how to keep us balancing on one foot, or judge the speed of a ball to know just the right moment to swing the bat and how fast. The fluidity and grace of the gifted athlete is not consciously willed or decided. It would be more accurate to say that it is tapped into.

Athletes sometimes speak of an experience known as being in the "zone," which they describe as a heightened or altered state of awareness.[1] Baseball players, for example, say that when they are in the "zone" they are able to see the stitches on the ball as it is hurtling toward them at ninety miles an hour. They also describe themselves as having a sense that it is not they who swing their bat. It is as if something else within them is doing this with an extraordinary power and accuracy that they do not understand or control. How are they able to do this? They have learned to achieve a more optimal synchronization of function between the forebrain and hindbrain.

When Jared was thinking of hitting a home run, he was initiating the movement of his arms from his forebrain. He was deciding what to do and when to swing. A split second later, via returning sensory inputs, the somatosensory cortex of his forebrain brought him a level of felt awareness of his movements. Based on this information, his brain made judgments about what was happening in his muscles, made decisions about what to do next, and sent readjusting motor commands to his body. But this pathway is slow and imprecise. And as we have seen, it is subject to the misjudgments of sensory feedback. Jared decided to swing hard, working his muscles too much. His timing was not good. He could not keep his attention on the ball.

Then I asked him to watch the ball and think of not swinging his bat. In other words, to stop trying to do what he believed he should do. When he did that, he turned off, or at least diminished, the impeding dominance of his forebrain. By focusing on seeing the ball, visual inputs were routed to his cerebellum. Together, these inputs enabled his *helper* to adjust the amount of work in his muscles and fluidly time their contractions to move the bat at the right moment and at the right speed. Now the bat found the ball, not because his conscious mind knew when to do it, but because his forebrain ceased its overcontrol and allowed his *helper* to play its part. I did not instruct Jared in the right way to swing his bat. I taught him to think in a way that helped him to achieve a better synchrony between the functions of his conscious mind and his helper. To put it another way, now each operating system was contributing to the task, appropriately and optimally.

When this improved synchronization is achieved, the batter says, "*I* didn't swing the bat!" This sounds nonsensical, but it is accurate. When we speak of "I," we are speaking of the self that we know, the self that is made real to us by the forebrain that is self-aware, that makes judgments, forms beliefs, feels, and decides to do a particular act. By contrast, when the helper plays a role in our movements, since this area of the brain is not routed through language areas of the brain, it does not speak to us. It does not say, "Okay, I'm here, now I will do that for you." Instead, like the athlete in the zone, we say, "*Who* did that? *I* didn't do that!"

Why does the forebrain become so dominant in our behavior, rendering the hindbrain, which should play an important part in our movements, less operative? I suspect that because much of our day-to-day activities are learned, and much of what we do involves keeping the body relatively immobile as we move a few parts (as I am doing now, sitting at my computer), we can get along well enough without it. We do not have to coordinate the whole of ourselves particularly well. Perhaps over time the hindbrain's contribution to our overall physical coordination becomes lost or weakened. This problem is misunderstood. It is not a problem of muscle tension, too much or too little, but a problem of malcoordination of the different yet overlapping systems of the brain. As bipeds, we are a composite of these systems, and we must learn to use them as a cooperative whole to achieve our potential for upright poise, skilled coordination, and self-mastery.

I like to tell students that when they use their prefrontal cortex to inhibit, they are preventing the malcoordinating habits of their higher brain. At the same time, they are allowing their helper to "step up to the plate." The good news is that if they can stop trying to do what they believe is the right thing to do, and stop trying to feel what they believe is the right way to feel, they will not have to concentrate so much or work so hard. With a little inhibitory skill—and a little help from their helper—the right thing will do itself.

In part 4, we will explore the second essential skill of the Alexander Technique, *directing*. If we can liken inhibition to cleaning up our cluttered mental house by throwing out what we do not need or want, directing can be likened to the new space that is recovered and within which we can move more readily.

But before moving on to part 4, in the next series of self-experiments you will learn how to inhibit, and to practice using this skill while performing a simple movement.

C and D

Intense feeling too often obscures the truth.
—HARRY TRUMAN

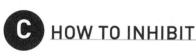 **HOW TO INHIBIT**

First, rid the mind of the idea of sitting down.
—F. M. ALEXANDER

CONSCIOUS INHIBITION IS an essential cognitive skill of the Alexander Technique. In chapter 12, I recount the story of my effort to unlock its mysteries. In the process I encountered four *mental pitfalls*—habits of mind—that stymied my progress. I have named these: 1) Chasing mental butterflies; 2) Feeling instead of thinking; 3) The loss of meaning; and 4) Avoiding "no." Eventually I taught myself how to overcome these pitfalls with precise mental skills. I have named these: 1) Quiet your inner conversation; 2) Turn on your prefrontal cortex; 3) Think with meaning; and 4) The positive "no."

In this section I will discuss each pitfall, and then follow this with instructions for learning its corresponding mental skill. Then, you will put your new skills together to practice conscious inhibition. I recommend that you read the entire section through first, and then try the experiments.

The First Pitfall: Chasing Mental Butterflies

One day I asked a student to say out loud the inhibiting instructions that I had taught him. I assumed he would do this with ease, but his halting effort told me he had not retained critical information. I was surprised. He had been coming for lessons for several months and loved them. What was wrong?

I went back to observing my own inhibiting process. Lying on the floor in semisupine, telling myself not to tense my neck, I discovered I was doing a lot more than that. I would begin by giving myself this verbal instruction, but then a new thought would rise in my mind and off I would go on this new tangent. Then another thought would spring into my mind. I would abandon the one I had been on and follow that. Then another would jump in, and so on. I was not inhibiting for more than the briefest moment before my mind wandered off into its reverie. I was not keeping my mind on what I needed to be thinking. *I was chasing mental butterflies.*

At the neurological level, this nonstop mental chatter means that we are using a particular area and function of our brain continuously and habitually. But neurons fatigue from constant use, making them less able to function. Perhaps that is what underlies the tense, pent-up feeling we experience after reading or talking for long periods. After all, there is nothing physically exhausting about these activities. Learning to rest our overly verbal mind is valuable in and of itself. Learning to keep our mind on what we want to be thinking is essential. Few people recognize mind wandering as a problem, realize when they do it, or know how to prevent it.

The first skill of conscious inhibition—quieting your inner conversation with yourself—gives your verbal brain a rest and allows you to keep your mind on track.

Quiet Your Inner Conversation

1. Lie down in semisupine. With your eyes open, listen to the silent conversation going on in your mind. Continue listening to this for

several minutes. Let your mind drift and let the chatter begin, and notice this as it happen.

2. **Ask yourself *not* to talk to yourself.**

You have to talk to yourself to tell yourself not to talk, but once you have given yourself this brief instruction you can be silent. You can also repeat this thought whenever necessary.

3. **Experience the silence.**

If you are successful, you will experience an absence of mental chatter while you remain conscious, seeing out in front of you, aware of both yourself and your surroundings. If you notice the chatter begin again, repeat the self-instruction not to talk.

Whenever you become aware of the chatter, repeat your self-instruction to stop. Success does not mean preventing this permanently, or even for ten minutes. If you can quiet your inner voice for just a minute or two, you are doing well. The purpose of this experiment is to become aware when you are talking to yourself and then practice choosing not to do it.

▶ **DISCUSSION**

After a short period of quieting your inner conversation, you may become more aware of sensory inputs: Colors may be brighter. Sounds may be more distinct. Feelings may be stronger or clearer. Since your mind is not preoccupied by self-conversation, it is more available to notice sensory information. You may feel calmer and more rested. Or you may experience some anxiety. If this happens, try this just for a minute or two at a time. With practice your reaction will shift. The silence in your mind will become familiar and you will feel more comfortable with the silence. Your aim is to be alert and conscious, seeing out in front of you, aware of sensory experiences and stimuli from your environment as you remind yourself not to talk to yourself.

Once you get the idea of this, you can practice silencing your voices anywhere, anytime. Walk down the street as you quiet your mental chatter. Do this as you ride your bike, or make dinner. Silence your inner conversation as you read, or as you listen to someone else talk—you may find yourself becoming a better listener.

The Second Pitfall: Feeling Instead of Thinking

Try this experiment: Silently tell yourself to relax your shoulders. Repeat this instruction to yourself for a minute or two. If you are like most people, your attention will drop downward as you focus your mind on your shoulders—trying to feel them, relax them, and determine if they are becoming relaxed. It is as if we try to shift our mind physically closer to our body in order to pay attention to it. What you have just done is put your mind on *feeling instead of thinking*.

To explain, let me return to the brain. Your brain is like a two-way radio. It has two channels, not one, as an ordinary radio does. Your brain/radio can *receive* signals (inputs) and it can *send* signals (outputs). It receives inputs from all your sensory organs, as well as from sensory receptors throughout your body. These sensory receptors transform types of stimuli—such as pressure—into nerve impulses that travel along sensory nerves, sending information to your brain.

Your brain processes this incoming data, *interpreting what these inputs mean*. Then, in response, your brain sends commands. These commands go out via motor nerves to your muscles, and also via the autonomic nervous system to your organs, blood vessels, glands, and so on. In addition, these commands may simply go to other neurons in the brain. This is a simplified model, but essentially these outgoing commands trigger some type of change in your behavior or activity. In short, when you are *feeling*, you are bringing your attention to information that is coming into your brain via sensory nerves. When you are *thinking*, you are sending out an instruction to make something happen in yourself. This may be an overt action such as standing up, or it may involve small changes of which you have no conscious awareness. For example, a neuron may fire to tell another neuron to *stop* firing. (Inhibition.)

Feeling is similar to receiving a call from your aunt in Florida, telling you a hurricane is on its way and the wind is picking up. Thinking is like calling your aunt back and telling her to stay inside and lock her windows. Feeling is a reporting in. Thinking is a command for action. Since your brain contains billions of neurons, you can feel and think simultaneously. But in order to learn to inhibit consciously (which is a type of thinking), you need to be able to shift your mind's attention from what is coming in (feeling) to what is going out (thinking). For example, putting your attention on feeling your muscles tightening is not the same thing as thinking that you want your muscles to stop tensing.

Feeling is relatively easy to understand and recognize. Thinking is more difficult. Neuroscientists have a lot more to learn, but on the experiential side our confusion comes from the fact that we use the word *thinking* to refer to many different mental activities: We say we are thinking when we let our mind wander; when we figure out a math problem; when we recall something that happened ten years ago; when we are asked to think of relaxing our shoulders, but shift our attention downward instead as we focus on a feeling in our body. These are all different activities of the mind. Our language fails to distinguish between them. But none of these are the type of thinking or *use of the mind* that is necessary for conscious inhibition. In the next two self-experiments you will learn to distinguish between the mental states of feeling and thinking. In the process, you will learn to make better use of a particular area of your brain. You will learn to *turn on your prefrontal cortex*.

Turn On Your Prefrontal Cortex

FINDING THE ATTIC

1. Lie in semisupine. Quiet your inner voices. Give yourself the mental instruction to relax your shoulders. Repeat this instruction to yourself for several minutes.

   Notice that your attention shifts down to your shoulders as you say these words to yourself, and your mind focuses on feeling what is happening in your body. Your attention has shifted down to your *mental basement*. You are using your mind to *feel*.

2. Quiet your inner voices. Ask yourself to let your attention rise up away from your shoulders and bodily feelings. Let your attention shift up toward the top of your head above your eyes. Repeat this instruction to yourself for several minutes.

Do not use your muscles for this. It should be effortless. You only need a few neurons—it is just a thought. Let your attention rise up. Think of rising up to your *mental attic*. By shifting your attention upward within yourself, you are turning on your *prefrontal cortex*.

3. **Shift your mind downward and focus on feeling your shoulders. Notice how they contact the surface you are lying on. Notice whether they feel the same or different from each other. Notice your shoulders in detail and for a period of time.**

   Experience this state of being in your mental basement, focusing on feeling.

4. **Ask yourself to see out in front of you and let your attention shift upward, away from your mental basement to your mental attic up above your eyes.**

   Experience this state of being upward within yourself, as your attention shifts up away from your body. You may become peripherally aware of bodily sensations, but these are not central to your awareness.

   What does it mean to shift your attention from basement to attic? Think of your brain as a house. Evolution has changed this house and expanded it over millions of years. Different sections have been added on to your brain, just as subsequent owners might add new rooms. Since you live in this house, you can choose to go down into the basement or you can go up to your attic. You can travel with your *attention*, shifting from down to up. This is important because different rooms—or areas of the brain—are suited for different types of activities. For conscious inhibition you want to think. You want to send a command to your body to stop doing something. To effectively think this, you need to recognize when your mind is primarily focused on feeling versus when it is able to think (or send) an effective inhibitory thought. To do that, you want to go to your attic; you want to activate your prefrontal cortex in the front of your head above your eyes.

5. **Let your attention rise up toward the attic in your mind. Then shift down to put your attention on feeling your shoulders. Shift back and**

forth in this way until you are familiar with your mental basement and your mental attic.

▶ DISCUSSION

The question I would like you to ask yourself is this: As I shift my attention up to my attic, is this a different experience (even if I cannot describe it in words or explain it logically) than when I am in my basement, focusing my mind on feelings? Can you notice a difference—not in your shoulders—*but in your state of mind?*

If you do not perceive a difference, perhaps your beliefs are getting in the way. Keep in mind that you cannot discover something new about yourself if you hold tightly to what you already believe. No matter how improbable this seems, ask yourself to suspend your belief. Think of yourself as an explorer, investigating an unknown territory. You have mental powers that you have never discovered before. This is your opportunity to explore them. Take time to experiment and learn new things about yourself.

Learning to rise up to your attic is not yet the act of conscious inhibition. It is learning to better activate the area of your brain that does the inhibiting. This is like making a phone call. First you must get to the phone. Then you can make the call. In order to inhibit, you must turn on the area in your brain that performs this function. Then you can use this part of your brain to inhibit. This is what you will practice in the next experiment.

THINKING FROM THE ATTIC

1. Lie in semisupine. Tell yourself to relax your legs, and shift your attention downward as you focus on feeling your legs.

2. Shift your attention up to your attic. Maintain this upward attention as you tell yourself to relax your legs. Repeat this instruction to yourself. If your attention drops down to your basement to focus on feeling, remind yourself to shift your attention up again, and then renew the thought to relax your legs.

   If you are like most people, when you begin to think about relaxing your legs your attention will shift downward to focus on feeling. If you notice this, shift your attention upward again and then tell yourself to relax your legs as you remain in your attic.

Your task is to tell yourself what you want to have happen in your legs *without shifting your attention downward to feel*. Trust that your mind knows what you mean by these words, and that there is nothing more you have to do. You do not have to put your attention on your legs and try to make the right thing happen. It is like mailing a letter: You go to the mailbox and drop your letter in the slot. Then the postman delivers it—you do not have to deliver the letter. Thinking a mental instruction or thought is similar. You do not have to take your thought of relaxing your legs to its destination— the legs themselves. Remain up in your attic, thinking the instruction. Drop your thought in the mailbox. Trust it will get where it needs to go without further help from you.

You can vary this activity by thinking about other parts of your body. Think of relaxing your jaw, neck, or back as you practice remaining up in your attic. Notice if you shift your attention downward, reverting to feeling the part of your body that you name.

▶ **DISCUSSION**

Conscious inhibition is a thinking act. This requires that you shift your attention up out of your mental basement and the apparent location of the feelings in your body. You must learn to *turn on the light in your attic*, the part of the mind that lets you be more widely aware of the whole of yourself and your behavior. This is like the difference between using a zoom or a wide-angle lens. Strong bodily sensations trigger us into zooming downward, overfocusing and narrowing our attention on our feelings. This distorts our perception, usually by exaggerating it. By zooming in on sensation in this way, we also block out other sensory inputs from our awareness. Rising up to your mental attic to turn on your prefrontal cortex helps to prevent this distorted perception. It lets you keep a bigger picture in mind; it gives you a more balanced awareness of the whole of your self. It lets you be more aware of your overall behavior, and to think of what *not* to do.

Learning to use your attic is difficult to trust. It is unfamiliar. It may not feel as though you are thinking or concentrating hard enough. You may not believe that this can be effective. You may react by thinking that this makes no sense. You may not immediately be able to perceive a difference in yourself. Keep in mind that your conscious mind cannot know the how, the when, or the amount of your thinking and its effect on your body. Your conscious mind can only know with certainty that you are in your attic, and thinking an inhibiting thought. The particular words that you use, however, and the *meaning* that you give them, bring critical substance to your inhibition.

The Third Pitfall: The Loss of Meaning

When my sons were young they loved to be read to. Sometimes I was tired and did not feel up to it, but their insistence was not easy to deter. Soon I would find myself sitting on someone's bed, my back propped against a wall, reading for long periods. Often they wanted to hear the same books that I had read a hundred times, and I would lose interest. I noticed that despite this, I could read perfectly well. There was only one problem. "I" was not present as I read. My eyes could scan the lines; my brain could interpret the letters and turn them into words; my muscles could move my mouth and tongue; but my attention was elsewhere. I could read aloud while silently talking to myself about making dinner. There was no meaning being stirred within me, attaching itself in symbiotic partnership to the words as I spoke. My words had *lost their meaning*.

It was, if you think about it, amazing. How could I be so unconscious of what I was saying, yet perform so well? Unfortunately, you can do the same. After quieting your voices and going up to your attic, and telling yourself to relax, for example, your words may have no meaning as you say them. Your mind may drift into blankness. If it does, your conscious inhibition will not be successful.

Words are simply sounds, sounds that are represented on the written page through shapes we call letters. We don't remember it of course, but we all went through a long process of learning the meaning of the words of our language. As an adult, you no longer give this a moment's thought. You just read. Or you put your thoughts into words and speak or write. But conscious inhibition requires that the words you say to yourself summon their meaning within you. You cannot say them blankly. This begs two questions: *what mean-*

ing should they have, and how do we think with meaning? We will explore this in the next two self-experiments.

Think with Meaning

THE MEANING OF WORDS

1. Say to yourself the word "hoicks." Try saying, "mohur." Repeat these words over to yourself several times.

2. Say to yourself the word "cancer." Try saying "snake." Notice if anything changes within you as you speak these words, as contrasted with what happened within you when you said the first two words.

You have probably never heard of hoicks or mohur, and so your response to them will be nothing or a sense of puzzlement. The thought might pass through your mind, "What is that?" or "I wonder how that is pronounced." As you say to yourself the word cancer, you might find yourself thinking of someone you know who is struggling with this disease, or you might feel a sensation of discomfort somewhere in your viscera. When you say snake, you might find yourself in your mind's eye seeing a snake, complete with colors and markings, slithering through the grass.

► **DISCUSSION**

What is happening in this experiment? The first two words hold no meaning for you. Nothing happens as you say them aloud or read them to yourself. Your mind is blank. Your body is unresponsive. The second two words, however, probably do have meaning. Meaning that has features in common between yourself and others, but also meaning that is unique to you and your experience. If you have had a close relative die of cancer or suffered from it yourself, the meaning of cancer will be chilling.

In sum, words are not detached from our physical self. They are not just intellectual abstractions. Their meaning has the power to affect us. Our life experience is kindled within us through our words as they stir something bodily, a felt experience in the present moment. This physical meaning is difficult to pin down. It is not just a synonym. It is not just a memory of the past. It is something felt and it is tangible. However, the way that we bring our conscious mind to bear as we think with words plays a part in determining the extent and nature of this impact. The best way to experience this is to practice consciously *summoning the meaning of words in your mind*.

SUMMONING MEANING IN YOUR MIND

1. **Choose words to say to yourself, any words you like. Say each word once. Then in the silence and space that follows, experience the meaning each word generates within you.**

Saying a word in your mind is like dropping a bucket into a dark well. Think of the word and then allow the bucket to return, carrying its fill—the word's meaning. You do not have to work at this. Your brain finds meaning by itself. All you need to do is receive it.

You might discover that what is triggered within you is a visual image, or more inner dialogue, or a vague, queasy sensation in your stomach, or a sudden laugh. Let me emphasize—do not look for synonyms. More significant is the ripple effect that subtly flows through you as each word is dropped like a pebble, a self-stimulus, into the still pond that is your mind-body.

2. **Lie down in semisupine. Begin by quieting your inner chatter. Then rise up to your attic as you keep your eyes open, remembering to be visually aware of the world around you. When you are up in your attic, say to yourself, *I want my neck to relax.***

Allow every word in this sentence to summon its meaning within you. Who is *I*? This is you—from your head to your toes and everything between. It is all of you, all of your past experience and learning, the whole of you in this moment. You *want* something. What is it to want? "I want my *neck* . . ." Trust that you know what your neck is and where it is. What is *relaxing*? Allow the meaning of this word to emerge within you like the bucket from the well. Do not be concerned about whether there is a change in your neck. Consciously think of allowing your words to summon their meaning within you.

3. **Try the sentence again. Say it slowly, with attention, with conscious awareness that the words have meaning and that your intention is clear.** *I want my neck to relax.*

Summoning meaning for our words is an act of trust. How does this happen? How can it affect us? Why does a word make us cry, grimace, or burst out laughing? How can the word "relax" create a change in the muscles of your neck? Neuroscientists cannot yet tell us exactly how this happens, but we can experience it and know that it is true.

Are these the best words for you to use as you inhibit? Try others. Experiment. Remember that the meaning cannot be forced, or made to perform on schedule. Repetition, lengthy but not mindless repetition, works wonders. So does patience. Say the words. Wait and do not worry. Allow change to take place within you.

Your objective is to become able to recognize when you are giving yourself inhibiting instructions in a blank, mindless sort of way, and when you are doing this consciously, with intent and clarity of meaning, presence of mind, and a genuine wish that their meaning will be received within you.

The Fourth Pitfall: Avoiding "No"

Thus far I have been asking you to say to yourself, "I want my shoulders (or legs, neck, etc.) to relax." I have been doing this deliberately for reasons I will now make clear. This is how I used to inhibit, and it is the kind of statement I often hear students using. Another common variation is "I want to let go of my . . ." (Name a body part and fill in the blank.) These statements all have something in common—as inhibitory instructions for telling yourself what you do not want to do, they have a serious flaw. To understand why, let us recall Alexander's story.

Alexander had a vocal problem. He noticed himself pulling his head back and tensing his neck. He told himself to pull his head forward, but he became tenser. Then he told himself what *not* to do. The instruction he gave himself became, "I am *not* going to speak," or "I am *not* going to pull my head back," or "I am *not* going to stand up."

If you decide to inhibit, it is because something is happening within you in the present moment that you do *not* want, or because as you tell yourself to do something (such as bend your leg) you start to trigger tension that you do *not* want.

In other words, something is already happening or is beginning to happen that you want to stop or prevent. Inhibiting is not just the act of doing something else. On a neurological level, inhibiting causes neurons that are firing *not* to fire.

Your self-instruction must be framed in the negative, because this is the language that means that something that has been happening or is beginning to happen should *stop happening*. To state an inhibitory command in the positive—"I want my neck to relax"— means that something that is not happening needs to happen. Something should get started. The positive form of the instruction is subtly telling you to do something. It is not another way of expressing the idea of ceasing to do something; it is asking for the opposite of inhibition. Stating the instruction in the positive almost always produces a subtle response of doing something in yourself, even though this may be slight enough that you cannot perceive it.

Since the positive language means *something is not happening that should be happening,* there is also an implication that you are not doing something you should be doing. You are remiss. You need to figure out what you are not doing and make sure that you do it. This can create a self-critical "I am not good enough" frame of mind.

However, when I give instructions to students that are framed in the negative such as to think, *I am* not *tensing my shoulders*, or *I am* not *sitting down*, they often object.

"That's too negative," they say. "Make it positive. I want to think positively. It's not good to think negatively."

For many people the negative has become synonymous with bad and the positive has become synonymous with good. Popular psychology urges us to think positive thoughts and banish negative thoughts. When students apply this attitude to inhibiting, it creates problems. You inhibit because something is happening that you do *not* want to happen. If you call the local Chinese restaurant and order chicken lo mein, and then decide you do not want it, what do you do? Do you call the restaurant back and say, "I *want* chicken lo mein?" No. You must call back and say, "I do *not* want chicken lo mein. Cancel my order."

Inhibition is a vital capacity of our organism for preventing what is happening within us that is not wanted or needed. Thanks to your conscious mind, you can recognize that you are doing something you do *not* want and take steps to stop doing it. When you are inhibiting, you are in a state that is characterized by the removal of something, or at least the lessening of something. Something is dropped off, left behind. Nothing is added. I tell my students in response to their objections that they have to get used to it. The positive does not always mean good. The negative statement is not always bad. Their meaning is confused and they can change it. There is power in the word "no" and we too often neglect it.

The Positive "No"

1. Lie in semisupine. Quiet your inner chatter and rise up to your attic. Say to yourself, *I want to relax my shoulders.* Repeat this a number of times.

2. Quiet your inner chatter and rise up to your attic. Say to yourself, *I want to not tighten my shoulders.* Repeat this a number of times.

    Do you perceive a difference in yourself when you think of relaxing versus when you think of not tightening? You may not initially perceive a difference. Perhaps you have already had the experience of your shoulder muscles letting go. You already know what should happen. Your previous experience assists you in giving the right meaning to your words, even if your actual words are not precise.

    Continue to experiment with steps one and two. Even if you do not notice a physical difference, be conscious of the different *meaning* of your words, especially the meaning of *not*.

3. Pick a different body part that you do not usually think about. Put your instruction in the positive: *I want to relax.* Then put it in the negative: *I want to not tighten.*

    For example, think of relaxing your back muscles, and then think of not tightening them. Tell yourself to free your neck, and then tell yourself not to tighten your neck. Do not look for a change in the feeling of your body so much as a change in the quality of your *intention*, that is, in the meaning of your words. If your meaning is clear, the effect will be different.

Did you perceive a change in yourself as you remained up in your attic thinking of not tightening? Being in your attic while repeating these words to yourself with meaning, especially the meaning of "no," means that you are thinking effectively rather than focusing on feeling your body and trying to *do something* to fix it or change it. At this point there is another pitfall. Because your thinking is becoming more effective, you may experience new feelings of muscular release. Then you may react by leaving your attic and going down to the basement again to focus on these feelings. Many of us have learned to be *sensation-tropic*—we are powerfully drawn to our bodily sensations. We like to focus on each feeling, scrutinizing its every nuance. If you do this, you will revert to feeling rather than using your attic to send a conscious inhibitory command.*

▶ **DISCUSSION**

It is vital to grasp the distinction between thinking of *doing* something (e.g., relaxing) versus thinking of *not* doing something (e.g., not tightening). As I have explained, for many people the words "no" and "not" conjure a meaning of "bad." Their meaning may be oddly unclear. "No" may be misconstrued to imply failure. For others it implies a state of emptiness or nothingness. Sometimes it is perceived as a kind of diminishment or lessening of the self. When asked to inhibit, some people think of themselves as becoming less than before: If I stop doing something, or if I take something away, I must now be smaller. I become diminished.

Ask yourself if this is your meaning of the word "no" as you inhibit. Does inhibiting bring you to a place that feels like a negation of yourself? Is there less of you in your awareness? Do you

---

* I am not recommending that we try to stop ourselves from feeling, or block out physical sensations. Feelings arise within us. We cannot control them, or how they are triggered. I am also not saying that feelings are bad. My point is that in order to inhibit we must learn to think, which means learning to send an outgoing signal to the body to effect a change rather than focusing our attention on a feeling, which is an input signal. Inhibition requires that we rise up to our attic and send out an instruction or thought, even in the midst of what we are feeling.

---

become tense, constrained, anxious, or worried about doing something wrong? This is not the meaning or purpose of inhibition.

By inhibiting you do not become diminished. It is not nothingness, emptiness, or failure. It should not activate feelings of anxiety. If on a subconscious level these are the meanings you attach to inhibiting—*to thinking of non-doing*—then you will create a quality of holding back in yourself. There will be a kind of shrinking inward as you inhibit, a diminishment or lessening of the fullness that is your self, a loss of energy and clarity. This is a most tragic outcome of your efforts! Paradoxically, when you inhibit, the self that is you becomes more. By removing your interfering habits, the living being that is you grows larger, expands; it becomes more realized. Your self is not made less when you inhibit. It is made grand.

Another misconception is that by saying no, nothing happens. But saying no does not mean "nothing." It means there is *less* of what you do not want to have happen. As a result, normal functions that had been impeded by inappropriate tension can work again. By inhibiting, you experience greater calm, clarity, ease, and more optimal functioning.

We need to give attention to the layers of meaning we attach to our words. Their meaning may affect us, even when we do not intend it. In the Alexander Technique, we say that we cannot change until we inhibit our old behavior to allow something new to arise. I would add that we are not able to change our old behavior until we clarify the meaning of our words, especially the meaning of "no."

Conscious Inhibition

1. Lie in semisupine with your eyes open. Quiet your inner chatter so that you can bring your attention to bear on what you want to think.

2. Let your attention shift up to your attic, activating your prefrontal cortex.

   This shifts your mind away from its focus on sensation and sets the stage for inhibiting.

3. Say to yourself, *I am not tightening my shoulder.* Or you might try thinking, *I am* not *tightening my leg.* Repeat these words to your-

self for ten minutes. Whenever necessary, renew your inner quiet and the thought of rising up to your attic, then repeat the thought to *not* tighten.

Since this is an experiment, you can try variations on these words. You might think, *Whatever it is that I am doing to my leg that I do not need to do, I want to not do it.* Or *I do not know what I am doing to interfere with myself, but whatever it is I want to not do it.* Whatever you choose, repeat the words many times to yourself without dropping down to your body to focus on feeling. Rise up to your attic and let the meaning of your words come alive within you.

If sensations of physical release come into your awareness, continue to inhibit. Whatever has been happening in your leg, whatever you have been doing to interfere in the whole of yourself, wherever or however this may be happening, consciously or subconsciously, at this moment, your wish— your meaning—is to *not* do it.

As you gain familiarity with these steps, remember to give the process time. Inhibiting can work wonders, but you must sustain it consciously with attention and awareness, meaning, and repetition.

▶ DISCUSSION

The first two skills you practiced in this chapter—quieting your inner conversation and turning on your prefrontal cortex—are like setting the stage. They create the scene or state of mind in which effective inhibitory thinking can happen. This is like walking into a room full of people where everyone is talking at once. No one can hear anyone else speaking. Then the room becomes quiet as one person walks to the front of the room and steps onto the podium to speak. Now you can listen, learn, and be affected by that person's words. By quieting your random chatter and rising up to your attic, your mind becomes present and alert. It is brought to attention. You have stepped onto the podium and the room is quiet.

The second two skills—thinking with meaning and the positive "no"—are the inhibitory thought. This is a particular type of thought. You are using words and summoning their meaning in your mind to tell yourself to *cease doing* what is not necessary, not wanted, not needed. You are delivering your message of prevention.

You can sometimes think in a manner that achieves inhibiting success without employing these four steps, but usually it is a hit-or-miss process. Sometimes it works and sometimes it does not. When this happens, you can lose confidence in yourself and in the power of inhibition. The steps I have outlined above, practiced separately and then in combination, give you the necessary skills for mastering conscious inhibition.

Ⓓ ACTS OF INHIBITION

> It is the means that determine the end.
> —H. E. FOSDICK

The self-experiments in this section continue your exploration of conscious inhibition. You will use your skills to prevent the habitual pattern of tension that is triggered when you tell yourself to bend your leg. Then you will inhibit to allow your *helper* to bend your leg for you in an entirely new way. You will learn, as Alexander described it, "to let the right thing do itself." But first you will practice two intermediate inhibitory activities. These are the experiments I gave Bruce in chapters 9 and 10.

Remember to give these experiments plenty of time. Enjoy the process of exploration and experimentation, and do not worry whether you are getting it right or learning it fast enough. If you give these experiments enough time, you are likely to discover that you have beliefs about yourself, your body, and how you move that you did not know you had, and that these beliefs have been leading you astray. I hope you will also discover that moving your body can be far easier than you ever imagined.

Stop Moving

1. Lie in semisupine.

2. Think of quieting your mental chatter and then rise up to your attic.

3. Begin to lift your left arm toward the ceiling, but after you have moved a short distance stop moving. Hold your arm in place as you

quiet your inner voice, rise up to your attic again, and think to yourself for at least a minute, *I am not moving my arm*.

4. Start to move your arm again, but a moment later stop moving. Leave your arm where it is as you think of quieting your voice and then rise up to your attic. Think, *I am not moving my arm*, summoning the meaning of each word.

5. Move a short distance again, stop moving, and think, *I am not moving my arm*. Then begin moving again, and so on, until your arm is extended in front of you. Repeat this process as you bring your arm down and rest your hand on your ribs.

Did you notice that your inhibitory thinking "turned off" when you began to move? The purpose of this experiment is to have the opportunity to notice when this happens and to stop moving at frequent intervals in order to restore your inhibiting thought.

Practice this go, stop, inhibit, go again sequence as you perform more complex movements. Try it as you play an instrument, as you walk, as you brush your teeth. Notice that as you stop, and think of not moving, you are able to release tension that has built up in your muscles as you move—even for just a short time.

Think of *Not* Doing

1. Select an activity that you know how to do readily, such as walking. Next, as you walk down the street, for example, begin to think of quieting your inner chatter and rising up to your attic. Then with conscious awareness of summoning the meaning of your words, think to yourself, *I am* not *walking*. Continue walking as you renew your thought of rising up to your attic and think, *I am* not *walking*. Sustain this for about ten minutes.

In this experiment you are thinking of *not* doing an activity *while you are doing it*.

What do you notice? Has anything changed within you? Does your body feel different? Is your state of mind different?

Let Your Helper Do It

1. Lie in semisupine with one leg bent and the other leg straight on the floor. Decide to bend the straight leg, and go ahead and do the movement. Repeat this several times—decide to bend your leg, and then bend it.

   Notice the habitual pattern of tension that is triggered throughout your body as you move.

2. Return your leg to the straight position. Quiet your mental chatter. Rise up to your attic. Without dropping down to your mental basement to feel, think to yourself with a sense of the meaning of your words, *I am* not *moving my leg*. Continue this inhibitory thought for about ten minutes.

   If a fleeting thought comes into your mind of moving your leg, see if you can notice the reaction this triggers in your muscles. When this happens, remind yourself to return to your attic while you think, *I am* not *moving my leg*.

3. Continue inhibiting, thinking of not moving your leg, and simply wait until your leg actually bends—*without making the conscious decision to move it. Wait and let your helper bend your leg for you.*

   You are probably thinking, *How am I going to move my leg if I'm telling myself not to move it? That doesn't make sense. That isn't possible.*

   These are beliefs. You may discover that you hold other beliefs as well. Perhaps you believe that your leg is heavy and requires a lot of muscular effort to move. Perhaps you believe that bending your leg requires pulling your thigh upward into your body and tensing your back. Perhaps, despite all you have read so far, you do not believe what I am telling you. Perhaps you believe that the mind cannot change the body. In short, you are learning about your beliefs—perhaps even beliefs that you did not know you had.

   Despite these beliefs, renew your thought to quiet your voice and rise up to your attic. Think to yourself, *I am* not *moving my leg*, and wait for your leg to bend without making the conscious decision to move it. What happens—in your body and your mind?

▶ DISCUSSION

You have arrived at a crucial point. You are up against not just the habitual use of your muscles but the habitual use of your mind—your *beliefs*. As we saw in chapter 12, your beliefs are tied to how you move. Because of your movement habits, you trigger accompanying sensory feedback. Your brain processes this information and forms beliefs about how you are, how things work, how it feels to do a particular movement, and how it should happen.

When you inhibit (in this case as you are lying on the floor and thinking of not moving your leg), your body is receiving new instructions that are telling it to *stop* doing what it has been doing. As a result, your body is sending new sensory feedback to your brain. (You may not be able to feel this consciously, however.) Since this feedback is unfamiliar, your brain does not know how to interpret it. Your brain does not know the *meaning* of these inputs. In response, your brain may *block* this strange data from reaching your awareness, or *take a guess* about what it means, or *invent* an explanation, or *misinterpret* it. Now you may hear your mind saying, "I don't believe this! This can't be right! This isn't possible!"

Your mind has created a belief about the meaning of this new experience: It isn't possible to do this. It is also doing its best to convince you of the *rightness* of this belief. And you will firmly believe that you are right, just like Betty in chapter 6, (You probably won't even speak of this as a belief; you will think of it as a fact.) If you give up at this point, your psychophysical habit has won the day. Rather than challenge your beliefs and learning something new, your mind has kept you locked in your old psychophysical behavior.

Even though it seems illogical, in fact one part of your mind—your conscious mind—can decide *not* to do a movement, while another part of your mind—your helper—does the movement for you. This unconscious mind is your cerebellum and hindbrain (see chapter 15). This is what I call the *helper*. To better understand this, think of your conscious mind as the president of the company. The president does not do everything. There are employees to help. Imagine that you, the president, want to send a letter. Do you type it? No, that would be inefficient. You have more important things to do. You ask your assistant to type it and mail it for you. In this experiment, by thinking of *not* moving your leg, you are using your conscious mind, your prefrontal cortex, to *prevent* your habit and to *communicate* with your assistant—your helper. Thus, you do not have to do the work of moving your leg. You can relinquish your forebrain's dominance and its belief that it must decide to do and then control the action. By inhibiting, you are saying to yourself, "Okay, I'll get out of the way. I know what I *want* to do (move my leg) but I am not going to do it. I am going to give the job to my helper."

Many of our beliefs about how we function are born of experiences we have in the physical world. For example, in the physical world you cannot lift a chair and *not* lift a chair at the same time. In the realm of the mind, however, such seeming contradictions are entirely possible. You can think more than one thought at once. And you can think of not moving and move.

If you stop deciding to do the movement, and wait instead to allow your helper to do it for you, your helper will do the movement differently than you do it. Your leg will move in a way that you—your conscious mind—cannot predetermine or preselect. You do not actually know how to move your leg differently. You only know how to do it as you have always done it. The good news is that you do not have to know how. Your conscious mind only has to inhibit, making the decision not to move, while asking the helper to do it. Your helper will do the movement for you as long as you do not let your belief that an experience, you have never had before is impossible stand in the way.

Let Go of Belief

1. Lie in semisupine with one leg straight. Take time to quiet your inner voice. Think of rising up to your attic, turning on your prefrontal cortex. Then think, *I am* not *moving my leg*. Continue thinking of not moving your leg in this way for at least ten minutes. Your task is to inhibit moving your leg as you wait for your helper to move your leg for you.

    Remember that you do not want to decide to move your leg, and you do not want to keep your leg from being moved.

The job of your conscious mind is to inhibit, preventing your *habitual way of moving*. It is the job of your unconscious mind—your helper—to move your leg for you.

If you find this difficult, do not be discouraged. *It requires a lot of repetition, patience, and time.* Whatever happens, you will be learning new and interesting things about yourself. The chief obstacle to change is the beliefs that underlie our habitual behavior. In order to change, we must inhibit our beliefs. This requires, however, that we discover what our beliefs are. Alexander said that beneath every misuse is an erroneous belief. These experiments are designed to let you discover your beliefs—and the fact of their hold over your behavior—as well as to learn how to use your helper. (It may be helpful to repeat the self-experiments in sections C and D, and to reread chapter 12.)

If you begin to have success, you will probably notice that a moment after you begin to move your leg, you abandon your conscious inhibition and jump down into your mental basement to feel. Your mind has become distracted by the sensations arising within your body as your leg moves. As you continue to practice this experiment, remind yourself to sustain your attention up in your attic and to sustain your thought of not moving your leg *throughout the entire time that your leg is moving.* Your habitual behaviors will not change if you inhibit before you begin to move but then abandon this new thinking as soon as you start.

As you learn to inhibit and change how you perform this simple leg movement, think of other ways to apply your skill. Use your inhibition not only to prevent unwanted movement patterns but to prevent unwanted behavior and unnecessary emotional reactions, *and to let go of beliefs.*

▶ DISCUSSION

For many students, these experiments strain the limits of their beliefs—not just about how they move, but about themselves. They find it almost intolerable to lie in semisupine telling themselves they are not moving their leg while waiting for something else—they know not what—to move the leg. You may experience this difficulty, too. Do not give up. Reread these instructions. Do not expect it to happen the first or the twentieth time you try it. When it does happen—when your leg does move without your decision to move it—I predict you will find yourself thinking, *"I didn't do that! How did that happen?"* (Remember Jared's experience in chapter 13.)

You will also experience your leg moving differently, with much less tension in your entire body. Your leg will feel weightless, as if it has moved itself. When this happens, you have rerouted your thought along a different pathway. Instead of using your *front stair-case,* going directly from forebrain to muscle, you have rerouted your thought from forebrain to hindbrain to muscle. You have used your *back staircase.*

In sum, it is not the job of your conscious mind to know how you move or to make a particular movement happen the right way. It is your conscious mind's job to prevent interference—both physical and mental—and so to allow your hindbrain to play its part. Your forebrain and hindbrain have different but overlapping responsibilities. To play a piece of music, the members of an orchestra must agree to play the same piece, follow the conductor's tempo, begin and stop at the right times, and play the correct notes. Similarly, the different functions of your brain must work together. The conscious mind has an important role to play in your behavior. It too often plays an interfering and domineering role. By stepping out of the way (inhibiting) and allowing your hindbrain (helper) to assist, you can make beautiful music.

SPACE AND DIRECTION

OUR HIDDEN SENSE

16

Fewer Words, More Space

The BRAIN is wider than the sky—
—EMILY DICKINSON

I BEGAN STUDYING the Alexander Technique during my senior year in college. In those early lessons, as my body opened and released into newfound freedom, I remember thinking I had been lost in the forest and had found my way home. Later, during my teacher training with Judith Leibowitz in New York City, my experience felt more like listening to Glenn Gould playing a Bach fugue. Gould's playing always seemed to reconfigure my nervous system, and Judy's hands did the same.

The many lessons I had with Judy over the years have blurred into a single, jumbo lesson in my mind. My most distinct memory is of Judy telling me to think "Alexander's directions": *to think of letting my neck be free, to let my head go forward and up from the top of my spine, to let my back lengthen and widen, to think of my knees going forward.* Throughout the training the exact purpose of these words remained elusive, but periodically I did something right and Judy's eyes would gleam in satisfaction. With her instruction, my body seemed to let loose and float up from the chair as if filled with helium.

But at home it did not happen. I could not reproduce the effect. As I observed my teachers and experienced their hands, it was clear that directing did something special for them that my own efforts could not replicate.

What was it?

Dutifully I repeated Alexander's directions. Then, instead of thinking the directions, I imagined a bubble floating upward, or a magical string pulling my head toward the sky. I gave up saying the words. I tried keeping a vigilant eye on my body to ensure that all its parts stayed in the right place. But no matter what I did, it never seemed quite right.

Finally, after years of experimenting, I solved the mystery. It was not impenetrable after all. I can now think these words in my mind in a way that consistently produces expansion and lightness in my body and a smoother, easier way of moving. What turned the tide? To tell the truth, it all began with some simple observations.

When my son Jules was five years old, I enrolled him in a gymnastics class. I was curious to see how the instructor would handle a large group of five-year-old boys, so on the first day I watched the class. Near the end of the hour he asked them to watch as he demonstrated a cartwheel. Then he asked them to try it. I remember being surprised that he was asking five-year-olds to do cartwheels. As I watched, my thinking seemed to bear me out. One by one, each child put his arms high in the air and leaned sideward to put his hands down on the mat. Then his legs buckled before he could get his feet off the ground, and he fell in a heap. A few managed to straighten their arms and get their feet briefly into the air, but their legs were lopsided and soon their arms folded as they, too, collapsed on the mat.

Then it was Jules's turn. I watched my son with interest. Jules raised his hands over his head, took a step, pushed off with his foot while keeping his body straight, cantilevered over onto each hand in its turn while keeping his arms extended. Each straight leg followed into the air like spokes. His body continued its revolution in space as each foot returned to the mat, body following, arms resuming their original position overhead. He looked like a windmill. The instructor smiled at Jules and said, "Good job!" In response my son wore a blank look as if to say, "What'd I do?"

This story illustrates an important difference between natural athletes and the rest of us. Like the other students in Jules's class, most of us become *disoriented* when our head moves away from the vertical. We lose our bearings, becoming unable to coordinate or balance our body as we move. Like a deer in the headlights, crucial operating systems in our brain shut down. Jules was a member of the minority—the kids who are a gymnastic instructor's dream. They love to be upside down and spinning, the faster the better. They do not become confused or disoriented. They are able to make the parts of their body go where they want them to go as they move through space, upside down or right side up.

Did you ever observe a gymnast flying around the high bar or vaulting off the sawhorse? Did you ever wonder how they *orient* themselves as they are flying through space? They not only orient themselves visually to a spot on the ground where they want to land. They orient the whole of themselves as they are moving, each part in relation to each other and in relation to the whole body, to the space around them and to the ground. Every body part moves in the *direction* in which it is *aimed*.

But what was it that enabled my five-year-old to do this?

I had no answers. Then another subject for observation entered my life. I began to spend long periods watching Cleo, my beloved standard poodle.

CLEO

Cleo arrived at our house as a twelve-week-old puppy with long, silky, blue-black hair that rippled in waves as she moved. All puppies are adorable, but Cleo had two special qualities. First, when you picked her up she did not stiffen and squirm, resisting support and pushing to be released like most dogs. She would let go of her body and melt in your arms no matter how tenuous the hold. My kids would carry her upside down, spin her around, and play with her. She not only had infinite patience, she had extraordinary inhibition. Cleo did not react. It was fascinating to see.

As amazing as this was, it was more amazing to watch her move. Opening the door each morning, I marveled as Cleo raced out the door and leaped over the steps, barely touching them. With her puppy's enthusiasm for the new world, Cleo flew across the yard. Everybody who saw her remarked on her elegant coordination, especially when for no apparent reason she released her body as if it were a coiled spring and propelled herself into the air, each leg spreading, her body wingless but airborne. There was seldom an obstacle in her path necessitating such a leap; it seemed only the spontaneous eruption of joy that sent her into flight. Equally surprising was how she landed. She never seemed concerned about her feet reaching the ground, which foot should land first, or even where the ground was. Her legs extended and caught her body with perfectly timed precision.

How does she do it?

I often took Cleo for long walks at night. Sometimes there was no moon or stars, and wandering down back roads we found ourselves in total darkness. As we approached a storm grate, I noticed that Cleo never failed to avoid it. Reputedly dogs have worse vision than humans, yet Cleo always saw the grate and circumnavigated it in advance. One night I tried an experiment. Before we neared the grate I talked to her, and made her look up at me so I was sure she was unable to see it. Despite my distractions and the darkness, Cleo avoided the grate. I tried the same experiment again and again. The result was always the same.

How does she remain alert to everything around her, even in the darkness and as I distract her?

I pondered these questions often as I lay on my back on the living room floor, Cleo in her favorite place tucked into a curl at my side, her nose resting on my ribs, her black eyes peering into mine.

One day I was watching Cleo as she sat at the bay window in the living room taking in the sights and sounds of the neighborhood. Then a squirrel ran across the neighbor's lawn. In an instant her head adjusted forward and up on the top of her neck. In the next moment her spine lengthened and her muscle tone increased as she extended her limbs and rose to standing, smoothly and effortlessly. All the while her mind remained focused on the squirrel, ears perked forward, vibrantly alert. (If she had been outdoors, she would have followed this with a burst of motion carrying her away in pursuit of her quarry like a popped champagne cork.)

What started this chain of events?

Cleo saw the squirrel. It was the visual stimulus that changed her mental state. This created an *intention* to act as she focused her attention on the squirrel. A split second later followed the slight adjustment of her head, followed by her rise to standing.

Was directing perhaps more an act of the mind than of the musculature? What might distinguish Cleo's mind from my own?

Surely Cleo was not telling herself how to stand, or where to place each leg as she landed, or which muscles to use and when. This was an interesting twist. We are accustomed to presuming our inherent superiority over the rest of the animal kingdom, but now I found myself wondering what Cleo's brain might be doing *better* than my own. Perhaps in acquiring our supposed superiority, we had lost something.

What is the chief feature of our so-called mental superiority?

One answer came back to me, again and again, like a bell's peal—language. Words. Other animals do not think with words as we do. They use body movement and sound to communicate specific, literal meanings in the present moment, but they cannot assign abstract meaning to sounds, or turn sounds into written words, or use words in an organized and complex syntax conveying past and future and conditional tenses, imagined events, complexly calculated suppositions.

Perhaps, in acquiring language and giving so much of our mental capacity over to it, were we diminishing something within ourselves?

Since Cleo's brain did not possess language, I decided to try being like her. I assigned myself the task of taking her for walks while enforcing my own inner verbal moratorium. No mental chattering to myself. No silent conversations. Happily taking in the smells all around her as we walked, Cleo was, of course, oblivious to my internal machinations. I did not have her nose for attending to aromas, but in the interval afforded me by this new mental silence I began to notice odd moments when, deprived of its usual preoccupation with words, my mind seemed to shift into a kind of bas-relief. A sense of space arose in my skull. I felt like one of those greeting cards that are cleverly cut so when you open it small figures rise up out of the flatness. There was a new and unfamiliar sense of spaciousness inside my head.

After further experimenting, I discovered that all use of words— reading, writing, talking to myself, speaking out loud, listening to others talk—triggered me into what I now thought of as my "flat mental landscape." I noticed this also included a downward movement of my eyes, as if I had to stop seeing out in front of me in order to think verbally. But each time I stopped this silent verbal activity in myself and waited, my mind shifted gears and this new mental expansion returned.

What is this odd sense of cranial roominess?

I often spent time lying on my back in semisupine in my teaching room, resting, waiting for a student to arrive, thinking Alexander's directions to myself. Now I became aware that, whenever I did this, my sense of mental space disappeared. I began to wonder if it was possible to think these verbal instructions while maintaining this sense of space in my mind. They seemed to be mutually exclusive. What did it mean, then, to "think the directions" as I so often heard it called? In fact, I heard this phrase so frequently I had not given it a second thought. Familiarity does not always convey understanding.

Why did Alexander use the word "direction?"

I got out my *Merriam-Webster's Collegiate Dictionary*. The first definition was a type of instruction, a "guidance or supervision of action or conduct." It could refer to instructions to be followed. This had always been my assumption. But as I read further, the fourth definition caught my eye: "The line or course on which something is moving or is aimed to move, or along which something is pointing or facing."

Could "thinking the directions" refer to a spatial orientation conceived within the mind, something akin to what I had discovered when I walked with Cleo?

My previous exploration into inhibition had helped me to understand that saying the names of parts of my body caused my attention to shift out of my attic and down toward my body as I focused on bodily sensations. I decided to experiment by omitting the nouns in Alexander's directions—the names of the specific body parts—and just to think of the directions themselves. I changed "head forward and up" to "forward and up." Merriam-Webster's definition kept returning to my mind: "The line or course on which something is moving or is aimed to move . . ." For something to move, I thought, space is required.

With my new ability to create space in my mind, could I think in a particular spatial direction? Forward and up was a spatial direction in the sense of the dictionary definition, but which way was it exactly?

I had no answer. There was a wide range of angular possibilities. But freed from the distraction of trying to do something to my head, and trying to notice if my head was moving and changing as I thought it should, I noticed that the words forward and up were decidedly unclear in my mind. My concept seemed to have more of a forward component than an upward component. When I tried sitting in a chair and thinking forward and up, my torso leaned forward and down. Try as I might, I could not conceive of a more vertical direction of forward and up. I decided instead to think each direction one at a time.

Which way was up?

This seemed clearer, although occasionally my thought of up seemed to list backward like a tall, top-heavy amaryllis leaning perilously in its pot. I tried putting the "forward" back into my up, but my eyes kept drooping downward. I seemed to be trying to move forward, rather than *thinking* in the *direction* forward. Since I could not think the two spatial directions simultaneously, I tried thinking the next phrase in the series, *back lengthening and widening.* Too complicated. I omitted the word "back." I tried thinking of *lengthening.*

Which way was that?

To my surprise, I discovered that the word made me think downward toward my pelvis, yet I knew with certainty that Alexander's instruction was to think in a headward direction.

Which way was wide?

Even though I had used the word many times, now I realized I did not understand it. I experimented with creating a sense of lateral expansion in my mind. After a few moments, my ribs moved more freely. This was an interesting change.

I tried thinking *knees forward*. The word—knees—sent me back into myself and made me shift my attention down toward my knees. I reminded myself instead to think in the direction *forward*. After a few moments this seemed to bring my attention more out into the world in front of me and heightened my visual awareness.

Like Cleo, perhaps, who never failed to see the storm grate?

Encouraged by these observations—even though they were mostly demonstrating how little I understood—I kept practicing. I pared the instructions to *up, wide, and forward*. I said these over to myself many times, one after the other. After a while I became able to think them together in my mind. I summoned their meaning in my mind, not as places for my body to get to but as spatial directions for my mind to aim toward. With practice, this process seemed to produce further muscular expansion and release. I seemed to lose the sense of the edges of my body. I seemed better connected to myself as I moved.

I thought the directions *up, wide, and forward* as I sat at my desk. My back did not fatigue. I practiced as I walked with Cleo and found my stride changing length, my gait becoming lighter and springier, my ribs shifting into higher gear to supply the needed oxygen. I practiced thinking these directions as I worked on my students. I felt less tired at the end of long days of teaching.

Eventually I went back again to the entire directions. Lying on my back with my knees bent, I went up to my attic, told myself not to do anything, and then thought, *let the head be forward and up*. I reminded myself not to focus my attention on either feeling my head or trying to do something to it. I simply summoned the meaning of the word "head," as I thought the direction, *forward and up*. Whereas before I had not been able to perceive any clear awareness of this direction, now I found it coming to me readily.

Next I tried thinking, *let the back lengthen and widen*. I changed this to *let the back lengthen* up *and widen*. I repeated the same procedure. I stopped trying to do something to my back, or trying to feel particular changes in my body. I thought the meaning of the word "back" and then the directions *up* toward my head, and *wide*.

Next I thought, *let the knees release forward*. The knees themselves were not important, I reminded myself. I thought up to my attic, and then I thought in a *forward* direction. Next I repeated the whole series. As I did this my breathing changed again. My eyes focused better. I felt more expansive, less constrained, more "up" physically as well as mentally.

When I thought these directions as I tried sitting down and standing up from a chair, new patterns of movement emerged without my conscious mind trying to instill a right way of moving. It was similar to the changes I had experienced while inhibiting, but there was something more. I sensed myself as more whole. I moved with a greater integration among the many parts of myself.

After a while I found that something different was simply operating within me. I did not have to keep saying the words. Some sort of spatial awareness was more consistently present. I thought of myself as having an imaginary gyroscope in my brain that spun simultaneously in three dimensions, giving me an ability to orient the movements of my body to the space around me. I was pleased by these discoveries but could not help wondering if it was really what Alexander had meant by directing. I needed more evidence.

What if I were to teach this spatial thinking to my students and notice what changes it produced in them?

One day as I was teaching, an idea sprang to mind. I summoned my courage and asked my student who was lying in semisupine to keep her eyes open and seeing out in front of her. Then I asked her to imagine in her mind's eye a flat piece of paper.

"Can you see a piece of paper in your mind, sort of eight and a half by eleven?"

"Got it," she said.

"Now, can you use your imagination and turn this flat piece of paper that is in your mind's eye into a cube or a box? Can you see it acquire depth, three-dimensionality?" As I watched my student's face I had the sense that in some inexplicable way I could actually see when she was thinking this.

Just as I was discounting this idea as sheer impossibility my student said, "Yeah, I've got it."

Probably made a good guess, I thought.

"Is there something about your state of mind that is different now, when you're thinking of this three-dimensional cube, from before, when you were thinking of a flat piece of paper?" I asked.

"Definitely," she said, with a tone of voice that told me she was intrigued.

I was intrigued myself. I decided to continue our experiment. "Now erase the cube in your mind and we'll try something different. If I ask you to think in the direction *up*—toward the top of your head, similar to the way that you were thinking of the spatial dimensions of the cube a moment ago—can you do that? Can you be aware of the direction that is up toward the top of your head and even beyond it?" I watched closely. Again I had the distinct sense I knew when my student was thinking this direction, and again she announced her success shortly afterward.

"Right," I said, "How about wide? What is it to think wide? Wide means thinking of expanding out both sides of you at once like smoke pouring out both your ears." There was a long pause. Her eyes seemed to be focusing slightly differently from each other and her face, while not literally moving, was somehow changing. Some sort of quality of expansion appeared to be happening on the left side of her face but not on the right.

"What's happening?" I asked.

"This is weird."

"What's weird?"

"I can think wide to the left with no problem, but I can't get it on the right."

In that moment I do not know whether I was more astonished that my student was understanding what I was asking of her or that I seemed to know when she was thinking wide to the left but not the right, before she said it. Since I had not admitted that all of this was as new and experimental to me as it was to her, I refrained from expressing my astonishment and tried to maintain a semblance of nonchalance as I replied, "Okay, give it some more time."

After a moment she smiled. "That's better. I've got it."

"Now one more. Can you think forward? Think in the direction that is in front of you. Since you're lying down, it's toward the ceiling."

Another pause. Her eyes dropped downward, then they rose back up. I waited. Her ribs began moving more freely; her eyes appeared more focused. This time we both smiled. Neither of us needed to comment. She knew I knew she knew.

"Can you put them together?" I asked. "Can you think up, wide, and forward at the same time? Say the words to yourself sequentially, but maintain the awareness of each direction as you add the next one until you have them all together in your mind. It is like thinking the three-dimensionality of the cube without visualizing the object itself."

It is difficult to describe what I saw. You could not really call it

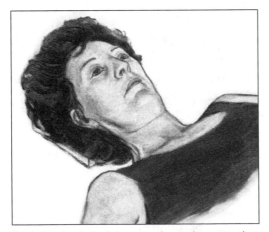

16-1. Student's facial expression as her attention is focused downward, feeling her body.

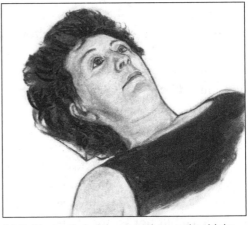

16-2. Student's facial expression as she thinks spatially: up, wide, and forward.

an overt physical change, but as before something seemed to emanate from my student. Like the pop-up greeting card, she seemed to acquire more dimension. She also looked more alert and less constrained. This was all the more fascinating as this particular student typically had an intense, cross look on her face, and she had arrived that day in her usual state. After just a few minutes she looked quite different (see Illustrations 16–1 and 16–2).

Not knowing what else to do, I finished the lesson as usual. Afterward, as she was walking out the door, she turned to me and said in a tone of surprise as a half-smile spread across her face, "I feel good."

MEGHAN

This experience so fascinated me that I continued my explorations with my students. One day not long afterward, a new student arrived, a young adolescent girl whose mother asked me to "See what you can do for her." The mother explained that her daughter, Meghan, had terrible posture and seemed depressed, tense, and uncommunicative. On questioning, I learned that my student was bright, and an avid reader who preferred to be in her room with a book than with friends or playing a sport.

After the first lesson, I could appreciate what her mother was saying. Although Meghan paid attention she barely spoke or looked at me. Her back was curved like a crescent and her shoulders were rounded; she held her hands tightly between her thighs. By the end of the lesson her response to my efforts was so minimal that I wondered whether teaching the Technique to a thirteen-year-old in a weekly, private lesson could succeed. And I wondered if it was possible to reach this very inward child.

One day after she had had about five lessons and we had established a bit of a rapport, I asked Meghan to imagine in her mind's eye a piece of paper becoming a cube. Then I asked if she noticed anything different in herself. She quickly nodded.

"Can you say what it is?" I asked with trepidation.

"I have more space inside my head," Meghan replied without hesitation. I was surprised that she perceived this so quickly, but I didn't say anything. I handed her a book and asked her to read to herself.

"Do you notice whether anything has changed as you're reading?" I asked.

Again without hesitation she answered, "The space inside my head is gone."

Since she was such a quick student we spent the rest of the lesson practicing reading while maintaining this new spatial thinking in her mind. At the end of the lesson I asked her to practice it during the coming week.

Over the intervening days I did not think much about the lesson, but when Meghan walked into my teaching room a week later smiling, looking up at me, and talking, I found myself speechless. Her manner of easy and friendly openness was so changed that I thought I had a new student. During the lesson she continued to smile, chat, ask questions, and talk about school and friends. I asked her if she had practiced her spatial thinking. She said she did and had found it fun. She sounded so comfortable that it did not seem to require further discussion, so I suggested she continue to practice this as she read.

We moved on to other topics, but for the next month I had an eager and interested student. Meghan arrived each week with fresh observations about herself, thought about her lessons, and shared with me the changes she was making and her observations of her slumping classmates. She was eager to change and seemed to enjoy her newly found sense of self. The lessons ended when her mother requested a referral for another teacher closer to home to spare her so much driving. I agreed but with regret. And I have not forgotten my young pupil and her striking transformation.

THE GOOD NEWS is that skilled directing is not a talent only the lucky few can possess. We can consciously learn to activate this capacity in ourselves. In chapters 18 and 19, we will continue to explore this skill, discussing where it comes from in the brain, why it is little known, and how we diminish this vital capacity within ourselves. In the Self-Experiments at the end of part 4, you will have the opportunity to learn to direct and to use this skill to enhance how you move. But first, in chapter 17 we will pause a moment to return to bodily sensation, and discover how our feelings can stand in the way of learning to direct.

17

More Problems
with Feelings

When the time comes that you can trust your feeling,
you won't want to use it.
—F. M. ALEXANDER

BALANCE AND COORDINATION are everyday words. But what exactly do they mean? More important, how can we learn to improve our balance and coordination as we stand, move, and perform all the acts of living?

To answer these questions, let us recall what we have learned: Our unconscious, psychophysical habits interfere with our loco-motor skill. And these habits are propelled by our mind's mis-interpretation of bodily sensations. Alexander termed this phenomenon *faulty sensory appreciation*. When he observed him-self in the mirror, he discovered that he could not reliably judge his feelings. Once he learned to inhibit, and so to prevent his habits of misuse, an unexpected result was that his sensory judg-ment became more accurate.

How does this happen? The brain is highly plastic: it can learn, unlearn, and relearn anew. As we move differently, new bodily feedback is sent to the brain. In time, the brain forges new mean-ings from this information. Like an infant learning to walk, we lay down new neurological connections and pathways as we change our behavior. But while this more accurate sensory judgment is vital, it can also stand in the way of learning how to direct. If we want to learn how to stand, move, and live with greater balance and coordination, learning to judge our feelings more accurately is not our goal—it is just the first step.

NATHAN

My young student Nathan has come to me for one reason. He wants to be a better baseball player. We have worked on his batting, catching, and running. Now he wants to improve his pitching. Joel, his father, a keen student of the Alexander Technique and a lover of baseball, has joined us for the lesson. As we walk into the backyard he takes me aside and says, "Nathan's strength is in the outfield. And his batting is doing great since you worked with him. But I don't know about pitching."

By way of response I smile and nod. "Come on out here," I say to Nathan. "Let's see you pitch."

Nathan is a quiet, sandy-haired boy in his early teens. He walks into the middle of the yard where I am standing and gives me a shy smile. His father takes up his position as catcher at the other end.

"Okay, Nathan, throw the ball."

Nathan winds up and hurls it to his father. The ball is high.

"Throw it some more," I ask.

Nathan throws again and again. The ball is low, high, wide, everywhere but in the strike zone. I ask him what he has been told to do to pitch. He gives me a long, technical explanation about his arm. It jibes with my observations. As I watch him move, I see that Nathan is focusing his mind exclusively on his arm, trying to judge whether he is doing what he thinks he should be doing based on how his arm feels as he throws.

"Okay, Nathan, here's what I want you to do. Forget everything you've been told to do with your arm." It's impossible not to notice his skeptical expression, so I add, "Forget about your arm for now, okay? You can think about your arm all you want another time. For now I want you to look at the glove your dad is holding. Look at the mitt. Don't worry about your arm, your pitch, or your form. Watch the glove. Don't take your eyes off it. Watch the glove while you're winding up, while you're following through and stepping onto your front foot, while you're releasing the ball, even after the ball has left your hand. Got it?"

Nathan wears an uncertain smile and does not look me in the eye. "Do you understand what I'm asking? It's like the batting game, but this time think of not throwing. Then think about seeing the glove."

Nathan gives me a nod as I step out of the way. He stands still for a moment. His eyes focus across the field on his father. He has lost the downward, inwardly focused expression he had moments before. He steps back, winds up, shifts his weight forward onto his left leg while keeping his mind focusing on the glove at the other end of the field. He sustains this as his arm moves past his body, bending fluidly and easily. The ball is out of his hand but Nathan does not drop his attention from the glove. A moment later the ball lands precisely on target.

"Hey!" his father yells with enthusiasm. "Wow!"

Nathan is quiet, but it is clear from his smile that he is pleased. His expression also tells me that he does not quite believe he did it. I repeat the instructions. He throws again—straight into the mitt. Nathan gives me an expression of surprise and pleasure.

"You see? You don't have to focus your mind on feeling your arm so much. Tell yourself not to do that. Your arm will do what it's supposed to do if you focus your attention on seeing the mitt. Think about where you want the ball to go. See the mitt. Don't stop seeing it. That's what's most important. Everything will follow from that."

⌒

UNLIKE BETTY, WHOM we observed in chapter 6 standing on one leg and taking a step, Nathan's difficulty is not one of excess tension and poor coordination skewing his sensory judgment. Nonetheless, feelings are at the source of his problem. Nathan has been given specific instructions about what to do with his arm as he throws. As a result, he has learned to overfocus his attention on his arm as he tries to feel what his arm is doing in order to know if it is doing the right thing, and to make correcting adjustments as he pitches. He believes he must focus on his arm in order to know what it is doing to better control its action. Nathan is operating from the common assumption that, by paying attention to the feeling of his arm as he throws, he will be able to carry out his coach's instructions and thus pitch more successfully. But by focusing his mind so exclusively on feeling his arm, he is diminishing his spatial awareness. Even though his sensory judgments are accurate, he is failing to put his attention where he needs it—to think in the right direction—in the direction that he wants the ball to go.

To offer an analogy, imagine sitting on an airplane listening to the engines hum and enjoying the view, and thus knowing you are on the plane. This knowing is well and good, and it is certainly correct, but it is not the same thing as sitting in the cockpit working the controls to fly the plane. In other words, the means by which we feel in order to know what is happening in our body is not the same as the means by which we direct—thinking spatially—to orient ourselves where we want to go. Being able to know what our body is doing comes to us from sensory feedback. But being able to skillfully balance and coordinate our body as we move in space comes to us largely from directing.

Correcting Nathan's problem was simple. He did not need lots of instruction. By asking him to focus on seeing the mitt, he restored this orienting mechanism within himself. I did not tell him to direct in precisely the way that Alexander recommended, but by bringing Nathan's attention to seeing the mitt he improved his spatial thinking. This in turn played a vital role in improving his overall coordination as he threw. Like Jared, who learned to watch the ball as he allowed his helper to organize and time the movements of his arms, Nathan stopped overconcentrating on feeling and deciding what to do with his arm as he pitched. By focusing on the mitt, he restored this mechanism of spatial orientation. In the process he experienced the critical difference between moving his body through *knowing-by-feeling*, versus *orienting-by-directing*.

Nathan's story highlights an important problem inherent in much of the instruction that performers and athletes receive. They are given a lot of specific instructions about what to do with specific body parts: make the elbow do this; put your fingers like that; hold your arm this way; bend your knees, etc. Although some of this is necessary to learn any skilled activity, it can also inadvertently teach us to fix our attention on feeling. The assumption is that if we focus in this way hard enough, studying, analyzing, and concentrating on a sensation (wrong or right), we will know what is happening, know the right thing to do, and be able to do it. Feeling and knowing are assumed to be the necessary and sufficient means for acquiring movement skill.

But remember that our feelings come to us via an input signal. They are messages that come into the brain because of changes in the body. Noticing our feelings is reassuring and informative, but it is a bit like a dog chasing its tail—focusing on our feelings makes us double back on ourselves. Sensations come to our awareness *after* an action has happened. As such, by focusing on a feeling we are actually putting our attention on an event that has already happened, albeit by a fraction of a second. By contrast, directing—like inhibiting—is an output signal. It is a command from the brain to initiate a behavior. To do this we must send a signal (a thought), rather than focus our attention on a result (a feeling). To return to our analogy, focusing on a feeling is like taking in the view from the plane. Directing is how we fly the plane, determining where we want to go.

Our common mistake is the assumption that accurate sensory perception is sufficient to change and improve how we move. This is what I call the "fault" in faulty sensory appreciation. But accurately feeling what we are doing is not sufficient. In addition to learning to inhibit, we must learn to direct.

Before going on to discuss this skill, we must consider one more problem that focusing on our feelings can create.

NANCY

Nancy, a lovely young dancer with wavy brown hair, a pretty face, and a willowy body, came to me complaining that she did not have good balance. "Can you help me with this?" she asked. Since then she has had about fifteen lessons. Today I have asked her to stand in front of the mirror.

"Nancy," I begin, "I'd like you to go ahead and stand on one leg. Either leg. Let me watch what you do." Nancy immediately lifts her arms away from the sides of her body, shifts her weight onto her left leg, lifts her right leg up in front of her, and points her toes. She

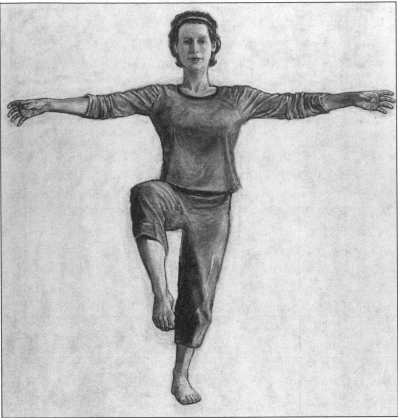

17-1. Nancy standing on her left leg and raising the right leg. Her facial expression is tense, the jaw is pulled back, and the neck is tense and stiff. Her shoulders, arms, hands, and fingers are also tense. Her upper chest is lifted, which means her back muscles are shortened and she is holding her breath. Her eyes are not seeing outward but focused inward on the feelings in her body.

stands like a rock. Not a wobble. I ask her to do this again, this time standing on her right leg. She repeats the same procedure precisely (Illustration 17-1).

"Okay, this time I'd like you to stand on your left leg and bring your right leg up in front of you as before, but then, keeping your right leg up in the air, move it in an arc around yourself. Move your leg to the side of your body and then behind you." This is a fairly standard ballet movement and I know my student understands what I am asking.

Nancy begins as before. But as she starts to move her right leg, slowly and deliberately, her standing leg begins to wobble. I watch the muscles in her left leg gripping harder as she tenses to keep herself from wobbling. It only happens more. Her eyes are down. Her lips are pressed together. She continues moving her leg in an arc until it finishes behind her.

"Okay, now put your leg down."

Nancy drops her right leg, lets out a sigh, and collapses her torso forward to stretch her back muscles. She has been working hard in the brief time it has taken her to do the movement.

"What would you say you're trying to do?" I ask gently. "Can you describe what it is you want?"

"Once in a while in dance class I find this place of balance. It feels so light and easy. I'm trying to find that feeling again, but usually I can't find it and I feel myself wobbling so I try to fix it. Then I get tense and frustrated, angry with myself. Why can't I find this every time?"

She wants to find a feeling from the past?

Like Nathan, Nancy is well coordinated physically. She also over-focuses her mind on sensation. Unlike Nathan, Nancy is not a beginner. She has spent countless hours in dance studios and per-forming on stage. Because of her experience, she is able to summon in her mind the memory of past feelings. It is as if she is remem-bering the view from another plane ride, when the plane was going somewhere else. She is orienting herself to a feeling but it is the memory of a feeling. As she moves her leg, she loses all awareness of herself and her surroundings in the present moment. She loses sight of now. Nancy's mind is on the past, hoping to recover a remembered ideal.

Dancers are typically highly aware of bodily sensations. This is like having 20/20 eyesight. People who are highly attuned to feelings often choose careers in dance, sports, or other types of athletic activ-ity. They love to move, in part because it stimulates powerful feel-ings that continually flood their awareness. Of all the senses, bodily sensation is their main course. They love the feel of their body in motion and can usually describe in great detail moments of extraor-dinary felt experience. Although it is all right to enjoy such mem-ories, it is not sufficient for learning to master complicated movements that require highly skilled balance and coordination.

Working with students like Nancy, who are professionals in movement-oriented disciplines, presents a special challenge. It is dif-ficult to persuade them not to try to feel as they think they should, wish they could, or remember they once did. When I ask them to inhibit their overfocus on sensation, they react as if I had asked them to give up the family heirlooms. My job is to use my hands to give them experiences of moving differently, in a way that is unlike anything they have experienced before, with better balance and coordination. Gradually they become willing to let go of their attachment to knowing-by-feeling, and eager to replace this with conscious directing.

18

Balance and Coordination

Nature does nothing uselessly.
—ARISTOTLE

IN CHAPTER 5, I proposed that bodily sensation should be recognized as our sixth sense. In this chapter I will discuss another sensory structure known as the vestibular apparatus, and explain why it should be recognized as our seventh sense. I will also discuss how this system functions, in order to shed some light on its essential role in our locomotor skill, helping us to balance and coordinate our movements, and enabling us to direct. I will begin with a simple overview of what a sensory system is.

Your eyes, for example, are specialized sensory structures designed to receive a type of stimulus (light) and focus this onto the back of the eye, where light-sensitive cells respond by triggering optic nerves. These nerves send their signals to the visual cortex located at the back of your brain. The brain processes these stimuli and interprets them. The result is what we speak of as seeing. It is a misnomer to say that we see with our eyes. We focus and transform light into nerve stimuli with our eyes, but we see with our brain. Similarly, the ears have specialized structures that transform sound waves into neurological signals that we can hear. The nose and mouth contain structures that are sensitive to air- and water-borne molecules that we can smell and taste. Thus, each sensory organ transforms particular stimuli into nerve signals that are routed to the brain, which receives and then transforms these signals into the gestalt of perceptual meaning.

The way that the brain does this, however, is neither simple nor inevitable. The brain learns to make sense of sensory inputs at critical developmental stages in early childhood. Further, each person's experience, training, and level of attention can alter and even enhance the brain's powers of perception. For example, professional musicians listen to music differently than those who have not received extensive ear training. Lack of sensory stimulation also affects the brain's perceptual powers. The brain becomes less attentive to sensory capacities that are little used.

In chapter 5, we learned that most of us have been taught that we have five senses: sight, sound, smell, taste, and touch, and we saw that this list omits our sixth sense of bodily sensation. It also omits the *vestibular apparatus,* another sensory system that is tucked inside our skull where it is hidden from view, positioned next to the inner ears on either side of the head. This sensory system is usually overlooked in discussions about our senses, or subsumed under the category known as **proprioception**, which is defined broadly as our capacity *to feel or sense our body in motion.*[1] But proprioceptive receptors are located in our muscles and joints, and so are entirely separate from and different in structure from the vestibular apparatus. And whereas these receptors tell us about the movement of our muscles and joints, the vestibular apparatus tells us about the movement of our head. Further, the sensory inputs from the vestibular apparatus travel to a particular area of the brain via a branch of the eighth cranial nerve. These distinctions warrant classifying the vestibular apparatus as a discrete sensory system, and numbering it our seventh sense.

THE VESTIBULAR APPARATUS (remember that you have two of these, one on either side of your head) consists of three tiny, narrow, semicircular *tubes* (also referred to as *canals*). Each tube is positioned in your head in one of three spatial planes: vertical (up-down), horizontal (side-to-side), or sagittal (forward-back). The tubes are filled with thick fluid. They are also lined with specialized

---

*This sensory structure is also referred to as the "semicircular canals."

cells with tiny hairlike projections. When your head tilts, turns, or pivots on your neck, the fluid pushes the hairs. In turn, these cells stimulate nerves that send their inputs to your brain. These hairlike projections are also set in motion as your head accelerates or decelerates, as when you suddenly change speed as you are driving. And they are stimulated when your head moves in space with your body, as when you bend down or stand up from a chair.

To give a simple example of this system in action, imagine that you are sitting at your desk and you hear a door bang open behind you. The muscles in your neck suddenly contract to turn your head toward the sound, so that your eyes and ears can better locate where it is coming from and determine what is causing it. As your head turns, the fluid in the horizontally positioned canals also moves. The hairlike cells in these canals are stimulated and send your brain information (along with proprioceptive receptors located in your neck muscles and joints), telling your brain that your head has *turned horizontally in space*.[2] Next, your brain contracts muscles to turn your body, *repositioning your body relative to your head*, so that you can readily move where you want to go.

The vestibular apparatus also includes two small structures called the utricle and saccule. These are filled with fluid, too, but suspended within it are tiny pieces of calcium called otoliths. As you move your head, the otoliths fall in the direction of gravity like particles in a snow globe when you shake it. The otoliths fall onto pressure-sensitive cells that trigger sensory nerves. As a result, your brain also learns about your head's movement *relative to the direction of the pull of gravity*.

Thus, your head's every movement sends your brain a stream of data. No other part of your body contains such a specialized structure for informing the brain of its whereabouts. We can readily imagine that as animals evolved, it became vital for the brain to know the location and direction of its head—home to eyes, ears, nose, mouth, and increasingly important brain. Seen broadly, the vestibular apparatus performs many subtle and complex tasks essential for an animal that moves in space and within a gravitational field, and scientists are still unlocking its mysteries. Fortunately, we don't have to wait for them to find all the answers. We can learn a lot about the vestibular apparatus by observing how we behave when it malfunctions.

Vertigo is a common malfunction of the vestibular apparatus. Its cause is not always easy to determine, but it can be caused by a virus or even by stress. Vertigo is often confused with dizziness, but they are not the same. You can make yourself dizzy by turning around in place for about ten seconds, which sets the fluid in your semicircular canals in motion. When you stop turning, you stagger from one leg to the other and the room appears to be spinning around you. You can prevent yourself from falling by putting your attention on the feeling of your feet on the ground (proprioceptive and bodily inputs) and by focusing your eyes on an object in the room (visual inputs). The movement of the fluid in your semicircular canals soon stops, and the dizziness subsides.

Vertigo, however, is something different. Instead of the feeling that the world *around* you is spinning, vertigo creates the feeling that the world *inside* of you is spinning. This is not like the usual perception you have of yourself in motion as you walk down the street, or feel yourself bending to pick something up, or the way you feel as your car accelerates. If your vestibular apparatus is functioning normally, even with your eyes closed you know that you are moving and you know where the parts of your body are relative to each other. But you would not say that your insides are moving. You have a sense of *inner stillness and stability* as you move, which are such constant features of your existence that you take them entirely for granted.

By contrast, vertigo creates the feeling that everything—inside of you and around you—is spinning. There is no sense of stillness at all. Sufferers go to bed and stay there, hoping to make the spinning stop. The slightest movement of the head reignites the feeling of spin. Strangely, this sense of spinning never completes itself in the way you would feel if you stood and turned your body in a complete circle. At least in my own experience, it feels as if the spin is constantly beginning—but never completing—its rotation.

We can learn from this that vertigo interferes with a vital function of the vestibular apparatus, which is to help you orient your body in space. Let me explain. Imagine for a moment that you are feeling hungry and decide to get a snack. With little or no conscious awareness, your mind quickly makes two assessments: your position in the house, and the position of the kitchen relative to where you are. With these *coordinates*, you can plot your route from where you are to where you want to go, and thus make your way to the food. Without knowing both of these coordinates, you could not orient yourself and make your way to the kitchen. Similarly, your vestibular apparatus helps you to know where you are in space and where you intend to go, and so to orient your movements purposefully in space as you move.

We can say then that the vestibular apparatus is a spatial-orienting system, made possible due to its sensitivity to both the *direction of motion of the head and the head's position relative to gravity*. For example, after you have been sitting for a while, the otoliths have stopped falling and the fluid in the canals has settled. There are few stimuli coming to you from your seventh sense. But as you pivot forward to stand up, suddenly your brain receives vestibular data that enables it to plot its coordinates for orientation: It learns the direction that is toward the ground by the direction of fall of the otoliths. By extension, it also learns the direction that is opposite to gravity— the direction I call "vertical up." (Illustration 18-1[A].) And it learns the direction of travel of the head from the motion of the fluid in the semicircular canals—the direction I call "headward up." (Illustration 18-1[B].)

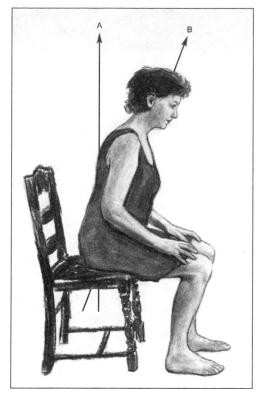

18-1. Orienting directions: (A) vertical up and (B) headward up.

As adults, we spend much of our time standing and sitting, which are positions in which our vertically positioned semicircular canal is aligned with the vertical up direction. But this is not always the case, as when we pivot forward to stand up or sit down, swim, or do a back flip. In these more dynamic activities our brain becomes a skilled mathematician, using data from the vestibular apparatus to calculate rates of speed and changing angles between our coordinates (the ground, vertical up, and headward up) to determine where we are, and to orient ourselves toward where we want to go.

This orienting ability depends on a fundamental capacity of the vestibular system that is widely overlooked: In order to orient ourselves in space, our mind must be able to conceive of space itself. Inputs from our three vestibular canals give us the ability *to conceive of three spatial dimensions, and so to conceive of precise directions within space*, as when we aim a ball before throwing it, or reach for an object on a shelf.

To experience thinking in a spatial direction, try this experiment: Simply *think* in the spatial direction that is up, toward the top of your head. Do not lift your eyes or move your head. Just think up. Do you notice that this requires a distinct awareness in your mind that was not present before? If you are not sure, try the spatial thought *downward*, toward your feet. Then think *up* again, and switch back and forth several times. (You will have the opportunity to explore this more fully in the self-experiments, section E.)

When you have vertigo, it is this capacity to conceive of three-dimensional space and to think in precise spatial directions that is seriously compromised. If you close your eyes, you cannot conceive of "upness" or "downness." Have you ever swum underwater, eyes closed, and experienced a moment of feeling that you did not know which way was up? This is similar to what I am describing. When you have vertigo, it is also difficult to decide to move a limb because it is difficult to conceive of space and thus to aim it where you want it to go. (You can compensate for this, however, by putting your attention on bodily sensations—by the feeling of your body contacting a surface, for example, or by feeling your body's movements, or by noticing visual inputs.) But vertigo seriously impedes our ability *to conceive of and to orient ourselves spatially*. In sum, if our eyes enable us to see, our ears to hear, our nose to smell, and so on, what can we say our vestibular apparatus enables us to do? We can now better appreciate that the vestibular apparatus enables us to think spatially, or, as Alexander termed it, to *direct*.

LET US TAKE a look at the role of our seventh sense in balance and coordination.

The vestibular apparatus is often described as our organ of balance. This stems from the 1830s, when a French scientist named Flourens made lesions in the ears of pigeons in order to test the ear's sensory functions. He expected this to cause hearing loss. Instead, to his surprise the pigeons staggered as they walked, traveling in circles until they reached a dark corner of the room. Then they sat down and remained there.[3] We can now appreciate that by deactivating their vestibular apparatus, Flourens gave the pigeons vertigo. This and similar studies are cited to explain that the vestibular apparatus enables us to balance. But this example can give us a flawed conception of what that means. We can form the misimpression that because the pigeons staggered as they walked, the vestibular apparatus was not performing its job of working the muscles sufficiently to hold the pigeons upright.

To better understand the problem this conception of balance creates, let me resume my story of vertigo.

When my vertigo is less severe and I am sitting in a chair, I can notice the moment when the feeling of spin begins. For me the spin is always toward the right and includes a slight rightward tilt. A split second afterward, my brain reacts to this *false feeling of spin and tilt* by contracting my muscles and pulling my torso to the left. Once I am actually leaning to the left, my brain compensates again by contracting muscles to pull me to the right. In short, my brain is compensating for my malfunctioning vestibular system by relying on inputs from my sixth sense, bodily sensation. As it feels me begin to lean, it pulls me in the opposite direction. But each correcting action is too large, and my body continually overshoots the mark. Since my vestibular apparatus is not functioning, my brain cannot conceive of the spatial directions toward the ground, vertical up, or headward up. In other words, my brain cannot orient my body to the vertical direction.

If I am walking when this happens, my gait takes on a lurching quality. First there is the imaginary feeling of spin and tilt to the right, then my muscles pull me to the left, then they pull me back the other way again, and so on. Like the pigeons, it appears that I am "losing my balance." But to put this more precisely, my brain is causing me to stagger because it is *compensating* for the absence of vestibular inputs, which are designed to help me balance by orienting my headward up direction with vertical up. *My problem is that my brain can no longer determine precisely where these directions are.*

Have you ever tried to ice skate, or stand on a skateboard? You quickly discover that your first challenge is to keep yourself from falling. These activities require a high level of balancing skill. You soon learn that to balance is not so easy, and that some of us (notably Olympic ice skaters) can balance a lot better than others. You also quickly learn that balancing does not mean holding yourself in a fixed position. If you tense your muscles excessively, you will immediately fall down. Your body must move in response to the movement of the "ground" beneath you. The more quickly and accurately that you can make small, rapid adjustments in your body as the many centers of gravity of all your moving parts shift and change in space and relative to each other and to gravity, the longer you will remain upright.

Now we can better appreciate that balance does not mean gripping our muscles, holding ourselves tightly in a position. Recall the example of Nancy in the previous chapter, who believed that to balance meant to hold her body still. When she began to wobble, she reacted by tensing even more, trying to prevent herself from moving. But holding our body tensely to keep from moving is not balance. Skilled balance means maintaining a condition throughout the body that is best characterized as having *a maximum potential for movement while using a minimum of muscular effort*. Further, for the vestibular apparatus to function optimally in helping us to balance, the head must move. Our seventh sense does very little to help us balance when we are tense and unmoving. If you observe a master of the art of balance, such as a tightrope walker, you will see that the entire body is fluid and supple, and the head in particular is continually moving, albeit ever so slightly, in order to continually feed the brain information essential for spatial orientation.

In sum, our seventh sense does not help us balance by tensing our muscles to keep us fixedly upright. Balance would be better described as an exquisitely delicate act of continually recovering—not holding—our uprightness. In order to achieve this, a subtle poise and mobility of the head on the spine is essential to stimulate our seventh sensory system, which sends its data to the brain, enabling it to know our spatial orientation—particularly the direction toward the ground, and the direction of movement of the head.

To more fully understand what is required for skilled balance, next we must consider the role of other sensory systems, particularly vision and bodily sensation. (Keep in mind that bodily sensation as I am defining it includes proprioception, the information we receive from receptors in muscles and joints that tell us about our body's movements.) To balance upright, we must draw from all of these sensory inputs in varying degrees and in varying proportions, depending on what we are doing. An important element in our ability to balance is not only what we do, but also how we do it.

Try this simple experiment: Stand for a while on one leg. Then close your eyes and do this again. You will find that it is harder to balance when your eyes are closed. Why is this? When you are standing or sitting, unmoving, there is little information coming to you from your vestibular apparatus. Your brain relies instead primarily on visual cues to orient you to the vertical upright position. For example, it can use the vertical walls in the room as cues, telling your brain where upright is. You are not usually aware that you are using your vision to help you remain upright, but when you close your eyes and stand on one leg, it is quickly apparent that you do. In addition, your brain uses inputs from proprioceptive receptors, such as the information that your knees are straight rather than bent, and from bodily sensation, such as the feeling of the soles of your feet on the ground.

In short, to balance well requires using a combination of sensory systems whose roles change depending on what you are doing. If you are running, your head is moving through space and so vestibular inputs play a greater part, especially as you increase or decrease your speed. If you are skiing, traveling at high speed down a steep mountain slope, making sharp turns and jumping over moguls, your head is constantly moving, accelerating and decelerating, as well as changing its position relative to gravity and to your body. In addition, your headward up direction is not aligned with vertical up. Now your vestibular apparatus plays a much larger part in maintaining your uprightness.

But, as I have said, balance is also a learned skill. It does not always function automatically or optimally. As such, your skill in balancing can be hindered by learned habits. For example, if you over-rely on your vision to help you balance as you ski down a steep slope, your torso will shift slightly back in space toward vertical up. This shifts your center of gravity back as well, which causes your skis to slip out in front of you. Or if you try to balance using bodily sensation, you will focus your mind on your feelings, judging their meaning and adjusting your muscle activity accordingly. But your reaction times will be too slow and you will tend to overreact. And if you tense your muscles excessively, fixing your head's position on your neck, trying to prevent yourself from falling by creating a reassuring feeling of effort in your muscles, you will prevent your joints from making subtle adjusting movements—especially movements of your head that are necessary for the optimal functioning of your seventh sense.

Remember Jules and his friends in chapter 16 as they tried to do cartwheels? Most of them collapsed on the mat as soon as their head shifted away from vertical up. To do a cartwheel, neither visual nor bodily cues are much help. You must rely almost entirely on your vestibular system as you direct your body in space, framing in your mind the spatial direction in which your head is moving as well as that of each of your limbs, while propelling yourself in an upside-down, right-side-up–again revolution.

Let us take a moment to summarize what we have learned thus far about the role of the vestibular apparatus in our locomotor functioning: It plays a role in our felt sense that, while we are moving, our insides are not. It helps us to orient our body in relation to our head as we move. It enables us to know the direction of gravity, the direction opposite to gravity (vertical up), and the direction of headward up. It enables us to conceive of three-dimensional space, and to think of specific directions within space, and so to accurately orient ourselves spatially as we direct our body's movements in space. It helps us to balance, a process of continually recovering our uprightness, especially as we move our head and trunk away from vertical up. We could say that the vestibular apparatus is a spatially orienting, righting, directing, and balancing system.

THERE IS ANOTHER vital function of our seventh sense that we must consider—its role in our *coordination*. Let me begin by clarifying that I am not using this word to refer to how well we perform a task: for example, how fast we can run, or how high we can jump. I am not referring to a specific skill in performing any particular physical activity. I am referring to a subtler action that should accompany everything we do as upright, balancing bipeds.

As the vestibular apparatus sends the brain its coordinates, the brain sends commands to the muscles of the neck and torso to adjust their

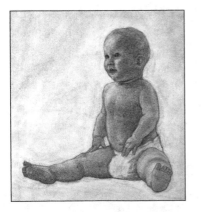

18-2. Baby sitting: the torso is balancing and coordinating upward; the head is poised forward and up on top of the neck; the arms and legs are lengthening away from the torso.

tone. Tone is a steady state of low-level activity in the muscles, which allows them to work for sustained periods. Tone is particularly important in the deep musculature of the torso. (This is the primary vertebrate locomotor system that we discussed in chapter 3) The vestibular apparatus sends inputs that trigger the brain to activate these muscles, increasing their tone sufficiently to support the entire spine, enabling it to maintain its upward direction against gravity. *In other words, the seventh sense assists in coordinating the activity of the trunk muscles to support and lengthen the spine in the direction of the head.*

In Illustration 18-2, we see this *lengthening coordination* in the baby as she sits. All healthy babies sit this way. They do not consciously decide to sit up straight, or tell themselves to hold their body up. The baby's torso lengthens upward as if pulled by an invisible string. However, this picture cannot show an essential element of how the baby does this: The child's head constantly wobbles delicately as it is poised on the neck. The torso also moves slightly at the hip joints. The resulting stream of vestibular data signals the child's brain to sustain the muscle tone of the deep back muscles to support the torso as it sits.

We can see another example of this lengthening coordination by comparing Illustrations 18-3 and 18-4. In the first picture, Burleigh sits in a state of relaxed and lowered attention. In the next picture, something has captured his attention and he has become more alert. Now his neck has moved slightly back and his head has moved slightly forward on his neck. As a result of these vestibular inputs, his brain has increased the tone in his back muscles to create a lengthening response throughout his torso. Alexander termed this upwardly coordinating mechanism a *primary control* within us that underlies and enhances how we move, helping to *coordinate* our torso in the direction of our head.

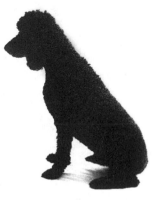

18-3. Dog: relaxed sit.

However, if you compare the picture of the baby with the pictures of John and Erin sitting during their first lesson (Illustrations 1-1 and 2-1), you may wonder if this is correct. Both John and Erin appear in stark contrast to the child. Neither of them sits poised easily upward as the baby does. John's spine is collapsed as he leans against the back of the chair. Erin's spine is stiffly held, compressing spinal disks and pulling her pelvis forward. Neither of them sits with either balance or lengthening coordination. Sadly, they are not the exceptions but the rule. We seldom see adults sitting with the easy uprightness of the young child.

What has happened?

In chapter 4, I proposed that the problem of our mind-body disconnection begins in our biology. Bodily feedback from our unconscious and habitual patterns of movement are sent to the brain, causing faulty self-perceptions and erroneous beliefs that skew our behavior, and for which we do not have an objective system of self-correction. In addition, our self-defense system is closely tied to our locomotor system. Long-term threat, often self-generated, causes the

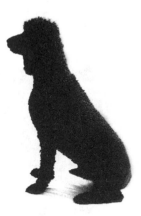

18-4. Dog: sitting with increased lengthening coordination.

amygdala to generate chronically maladaptive responses in our musculature, further fueling this cycle.

But we face additional challenges. Millions of years ago, when humans began to develop the capacity to think with words, there was no extra space in the skull for additional neurons to perform this function. What happened? Scientists tell us that prior to the development of language, we had two areas in the brain—one on either side—for spatial thinking. Apparently, one of these areas was usurped for language. Today we literally have less brain for thinking spatially.[4] Further, because we have a talent for language, we use it. Most of us spend virtually all our waking hours engaged in reading, writing, speaking, listening, or silently talking to ourselves with words. As we saw in the case of Meghan, this condition might be viewed as an overuse syndrome, creating a brownout in our brains: With too many mental functions vying for a finite amount of energy, each gets less. *We give our mind's attention to language, not to space.*

In addition, since most of us have learned unconsciously to maintain our uprightness primarily through visual inputs, our brain's attention to vestibular information is reduced. Have you noticed that children love to swing, and hang upside down from a jungle gym? Most adults feel nauseated after just a few minutes on a swing, and we rarely find grown-ups hanging upside down anywhere. By adulthood, we have become habituated to maintaining our head-ward-up direction aligned with vertical up. This significantly limits inputs from the vestibular system. Over time, the brain learns to make do with less and less vestibular information. But our sensory systems need to be used in order for the brain's perceptual powers to become finely tuned and highly skilled. Without motion we limit the inputs to, and the use of, our seventh sensory system.

Finally, excess tension—especially in the muscles of the neck, jaw, shoulders, and upper back—create particular problems. As Alexander correctly observed, because the vestibular system is sensitive to the movement of the head, the data it gathers can become distorted by overtensing and malcoordinating our head and neck musculature: *first, by fixing the position of the head on top of the neck; second, by misaligning the normal upright poise of the neck (which in turn also affects the head's position).* Trying to move efficiently and skillfully while malcoordinating our head and neck is like putting a rain gauge under a tree, positioning it on a slant, and expecting it to take an accurate reading. The instrument's placement and alignment interferes with its ability to function, skewing its data. Excessive neck tension does the same to the vestibular system. (Take a moment to review the illustrations of head and neck malcoordination in II-1 and II-2.)

How do we remedy the many factors that impede the functioning of our vestibular system?

First, it is important to increase sensory inputs to this system by increasing movement activity, especially movements that take the head and torso away from vertical up. Next, it is important to let the brain's overburdened language function have a rest by lessening our verbal activity. (If you have not tried it yet, section C includes a self-experiment for learning how to do this.)

The best method for remedying our unconscious interference with our vestibular system was developed by F. M. Alexander: First, his method teaches us how to reduce unnecessary muscle tension, particularly in the head, neck, and shoulders through conscious inhibition. Second, it teaches us how to develop our brain's attention to spatial inputs through conscious direction. Just as practice can heighten our other sensory powers—the ability to listen to music, to appreciate a fine wine, to observe the use of color in a painting—we can consciously develop our powers of spatial thinking through directing, thereby restoring and awakening this vital balance and coordination system within us.

19

A New Way of Moving

I'm not afraid of storms,
for I'm learning to sail my ship.
—LOUISA MAY ALCOTT

BRIAN

Recently, A MAN called asking for an appointment for his teenage son. He told me that Brian was a violinist and suffered from severe facial pain. The next week, when Brian arrived, I welcomed a tall, dark-haired, round-faced fifteen-year-old into my teaching room. When I asked him to describe his pain, Brian put his hands on the sides of his face, lowered his head, and grimaced. With this single gesture he drew a compelling picture of pain.

It soon became clear that Brian's jaw muscles were exceedingly tight, particularly on the left side where he held his violin. I also could not help noticing the look in his eyes. Teenagers often wear a sulky, "don't come near me" expression, but Brian's was acute. It was almost painful to look at him, impossible to get him to make eye contact with me, and a smile was a rare event. Despite his seemingly unapproachable manner, Brian's father assured me after his second visit that he liked the lessons and wanted to continue.

At Brian's next lesson I decided to take an unprecedented leap. Even though I had just begun to introduce inhibition and hadn't yet worked with him in the chair, I put him on the table and after some initial work asked Brian to imagine in his mind's eye a flat piece of paper. Then I asked him to imagine this paper becoming a cube, gaining another dimension. With some practice he seemed to be getting this, so I asked him to think up, then wide, and then forward. After about fifteen minutes Brian was thinking spatially with ease. I got him off the table and asked him to stand in front of the chair.

In previous lessons, I had watched Brian closely as I explained the basic concepts of the Technique. It was impossible not to notice that he had no upward coordination in his torso at all. His spine was so curved as he sat that he lost at least four inches in height. His neck was pulled forward, his head clutched backward onto his neck.

Today, rather than telling him about his misuse of himself, I stood next to him as I placed my right hand lightly on the back of his head and neck, and my left hand on his hip. Then I asked him to think again: up, wide, and forward.

Even after decades of teaching, what happened next took me completely by surprise. Something seemed to come unfastened within him as Brian's torso lengthened upward by several inches. His leg muscles released. Then he folded neatly at his hips, knees, and ankles, his torso lengthening headward, and floated lightly down into the chair.

When he was sitting in the chair with a newly upright torso and a head poised beautifully on top of his lengthening spine, I suggested that he turn his head to look at himself in the mirror.

"Do you notice anything different about yourself?" I asked.

Brian was silent as he looked in the mirror. His eyes were focused and bright. A smile was beginning to spread the corners of his mouth. He looked like an entirely different person. Then he noticed me watching him in the mirror.

"It's kinda different," he answered, not losing eye contact with me.

"Yes, it is," I said, smiling back at him.

I suggested that he practice thinking spatially over the coming week as he practiced his violin.

"Yeah," Brian answered, his smile stretching into a toothy grin.

Brian had no idea of the excitement I felt at his sudden transformation. The change in his upward coordination was a vivid example of the power of directing. I had not given him any explanation about how to sit, what to do or not do in his body, or even told him that I wanted him to sit. I had asked him just to think spatially, and his posture and way of moving was immediately transformed.

I have no doubt that after years of practicing his violin—bracing onto the instrument with a powerful clutch in his neck and jaw muscles; holding his head, neck, and torso rigidly in this position for hours as he practiced; focusing his attention narrowly downward onto his fingers and bow; worrying about incorrect notes and errant sounds— Brian had created the constellation of conditions that created his pain. But his pain was not his central problem. His pain was only the end result, the product of years of malcoordinating tension that locked his head onto his body as he focused his attention ever more narrowly downward.

This physical and mental compression had become so extreme that Brian seemed to be locked inside, as if backed up against an inner wall with nowhere to go. The sudden change as he shifted his thinking and directed up, wide, and forward was like watching someone emerge from a dark cave into the bright light of day.

BETTY, PART TWO

We return to Betty, whom we met in chapter 6. Betty was learning that she had a habit of collapsing downward on her hip and compressing in her torso whenever she stood on her left leg to take a step. I used my hands to guide her in standing more upright as she inhibited. Her torso coordinated more upward and she did not collapse. But Betty insisted this new way of standing felt wrong, adding that it felt as if her leg would not support her weight. When I asked her to take a step, she could not help reverting to her old way of standing, even though my hands were supporting her. Since then Betty has been learning to direct. She has been practicing this in her lessons while sitting in and standing from a chair. Today we are returning to standing on one leg.

"Betty, would you turn to face the mirror so you can observe yourself as we're doing this."

Betty turns toward the mirror. I look at her expression and see her concern.

"Okay, Betty, before we begin let's talk about using the mirror.

Looking in the mirror is difficult. We become critical when we look at ourselves. But in the lesson we're not using the mirror to make judgments, good or bad. We're using it to observe, to see things that we may not be able to feel. We're also using it to observe ourselves moving as we inhibit and direct. You want to be able to inhibit and direct as you cross the street and watch for cars, or wash the dishes, or play tennis. You need to be able to think and see at the same time. So I want you to think and keep looking in the mirror. Is that okay?" I add, inviting comment.

"Okay," Betty answers with a slight smile, letting me know that I have touched on a source of her anxiety.

"I'm going to stand behind you with my hands on your ribs. Then I'm going to shift your torso slightly to the left to bring your body over your left leg. As we do this, I'd like you to inhibit. Just think of not shifting your weight, or not doing anything. Think of not reacting to what is happening. I'm going to do the movement for you. You don't have to help." I guide Betty's torso a few inches to the left.

"That's great, Betty. Now direct. Think spatially: up, wide, and forward."

I watch Betty closely in the mirror as I am speaking. At the same time, my hands feel subtle changes in her body. I feel that her torso is coordinating upward and her ribs are moving freely. Her torso is balancing on top of her leg, poised rather than collapsed downward into her hip. She is light and easy to move. Nothing is rigid or held. There is no feeling of resistance, anticipation, or reaction. She is calm, balanced, and coordinated.

"Okay, Betty, that's good. Continue directing. That's it. You're balancing on your left leg. This is what we want. This is what standing on a leg should be—light and effortless. Now think of directing forward and take a step." As I add these instructions, I feel Betty's hesitation. Beneath my hands she suddenly feels hesitant like a child standing at the pool's edge wanting to dive in but suddenly afraid and drawing back.

"I still don't feel like I can stand on this leg," Betty says with a tone of worry.

I shift her back to standing on both legs and take away my hands. Then I walk around to stand in front of her as I speak.

"I understand that is how it feels, Betty. But remember, this is the part of your brain that judges this new feeling by comparing it to what it has previously experienced. I'm helping you to stand in a new way, so you're experiencing a new feeling that your brain doesn't understand. Your brain has to make a guess about what this new feeling means. And it is guessing that you can't stand, because it doesn't associate this feeling with the act of standing. But this judgment isn't based on an objective truth. In fact, it's incorrect. If you continue to believe this, what will you do?"

"I'll go back to standing in my old way?"

"You've got it. The more you focus on what you believe this feeling means, the more you'll revert to the old way of moving. I'm not saying that you should try to stop feeling. Your feelings aren't bad. It's just that the judgments you form from them might not be correct. You don't want to block out your feelings or your judgments, but you do want to remember that they aren't always right. Especially when you're doing something new, your judgments about what your feelings mean are unreliable. And they aren't a very good way to help you learn a new way to coordinate your body as you stand and walk. Remind yourself not to put all your attention on what you're feeling. Put your attention on what you're thinking—that is, inhibiting and directing. Can you do that?"

Betty responds with a nod.

I walk behind her and place my hands on her ribs again. "Think up to your attic and think of not standing and not judging your feelings. Then renew your directions: up, wide, forward. That's good, Betty, that's it."

I shift Betty's torso over her left leg. "Continue directing. These are spatial directions of where you're aiming toward: your head and torso are aiming upward, your shoulders are aiming wide, the leg you're standing on is lengthening, aiming toward the ground, and your right knee is aiming forward."

I pause as Betty stands on her left leg, directing. I observe in the mirror that she is seeing in front of her rather than dropping her eyes. My hands feel her torso lengthening upward, her ribs moving; she is balancing again. Then, without any change in this easy balance and upward poise, Betty's right knee, hip, and ankle bend as she steps forward onto her right foot.

This time she has performed the act of standing and taking a step entirely differently. There is no sideward lurch of her pelvis, no tilt in the torso, and no downward compression on her hip or hiking up on her bending leg. She has continued seeing out in front of her, attentive to the world around her while inhibiting and directing (see Illustration 19-1). I see in the mirror that Betty's face has spread into an expression of pleasure and wonder.

"I didn't do that," Betty says. "You did that. You moved me and made that happen. I didn't do that. I didn't do it." Words of protest and astonishment tumble out.

"What makes you think I did it?" I ask.

"I didn't decide to move my leg. I didn't do anything. It felt like nothing."

"I didn't move you, Betty, I didn't touch your leg."

Betty is silent as she looks down. Then she looks up and sees me in the mirror, smiling, watching her. We burst into laughter.

"You didn't move my leg?" she asks, still giggling. "How did that happen? I never move like that. It felt . . . like nothing!"

Betty's is the laughter of surprise and delight. Mine is of satisfaction. Another student has opened a door and stepped into a new world of mind-body connection and self-mastery. Betty is learning, in a way that no amount of discussion could persuade her, the power of bodily sensation to create false assumptions, wrong beliefs, and maladaptive behavior. She has begun learning to replace the old system of judging-by-feeling with the simple clarity of inhibition and direction. The many disparate pieces of her self become integrated, connected. She stands and walks with balance, upward coordination, and grace.

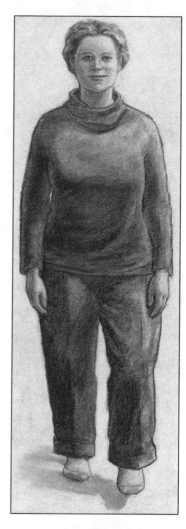

19-1. Betty standing on right leg and taking a step, while inhibiting and directing. Her torso is vertically aligned on top of her vertical right leg; her shoulders are wide apart and level, her arms hang freely; her facial expression shows attention, awareness, and spatial thinking.

⁓

IMAGINE THAT YOU are on a boat in the middle of a lake on a dark night trying to navigate, but it is too dark to see ahead of you.

"I don't know where I am," you think worriedly to yourself.

Then, in order to know where you are, you pick up a flashlight and shine it on yourself.

Of course this sounds silly, but in a sense now you know where you are. The problem is, you do not know where you want to go.

Now imagine yourself pointing the flashlight ahead of you. You can see some rocks and buoys. Aiming the light, you steer the boat around the rocks and between the buoys, and slowly navigate your way across the lake.

Shining the light on yourself is like trying to orient and coordinate yourself by using bodily sensation, focusing the light of attention inward upon yourself, trying to locate and know the meaning of your feelings, acting in reaction to how you feel. Shining the light in front of you is like orienting and coordinating yourself by directing—knowing the space around you and determining where you want to go. Conscious directing enables you to balance and coordinate your movements, and the whole of yourself, in space. This is the vital power of your seventh sense.

E and F

(E) HOW TO DIRECT

DIRECTING CREATES AN enhancement in our movement coordination beyond what is created by inhibiting alone. Directing gives us coordination and balance without loss of mobility. It creates strength without strain, energy without tension, and expansion without loss of focus. As we direct, we are both the being that propels ourselves into action, and the being that is acted upon. It is as if we become the pitcher who skillfully aims the ball and the ball that is thrown. I am reminded of directing's power when I watch a male dancer lifting a ballerina: She leaps into the air as his arms catch and lift her higher, carrying and directing her through space along the trajectory that her body has aimed. Through their pairing, she seems suspended in air for a brief moment of eternity.

SELF-EXPERIMENTS

In this series of experiments, you will begin practicing this skill by learning to think spatially, and then sustain this thinking as you turn your head. You will learn to think in a precise spatial direction—forward and up. You will practice thinking spatially as you think of specific parts of your body. Finally, you will put these skills together to think Alexander's directions: to let the neck be back, to let the head be forward and up, to let the torso lengthen up and widen, and to let the knees release forward.

Think of a Cube

1. Lie in semisupine with your eyes open. In your mind's eye, imagine a piece of notebook paper. Then imagine this piece of paper expanding into a third dimension—gaining depth to become a rectangular box.

    See the paper expand like a flat sponge absorbing water, so that you perceive a three-dimensional object instead of a flat one.

2. Shift back and forth in your mind, from the rectangular box to the flat piece of paper, then back to the box, etc.

    Can you notice a subtle change in your mind as you do this? It is difficult to put into words, but there is something different in your mind as you conceive of the flat piece of paper or the three-dimensional box. This is a fairly easy way to experience what I call *spatial thinking*. It is the capacity of your mind to conceive of three dimensions.

Up-Down, Wide, Forward-Back

1. Lie in semisupine. Summon in your mind an awareness of the spatial direction that is "up" toward the top of your head.

    Be sure not to lift your eyes, tense your face or neck muscles, pull your head back, or generate other muscular tension. Ask yourself only to think in the direction that is up, toward your head. This is not a physical effort. Let the word "up" summon its meaning in your mind. This direction is not a specific place that you arrive at. It is a direction you think toward with a sense of ongoing motion like a river flowing without end.

2. Ask yourself to think in an "up" direction and let the thought of this direction continue beyond the top of your head. You can have a sense of "up" that continues through and beyond your physical self. Have a sense of "up" that extends two feet above your head, ten feet, a mile, a hundred miles. Whatever you choose.

   This is an imaginative act—a thought of upward direction. Once the word triggers a sense of upward expansion in yourself, you do not have to keep saying it. Simply be aware that you are allowing this *spatial direction* to become enlivened within you. If you notice that you lose your thought of the up direction, just repeat the word again.

3. Think in the direction that is the meaning of the word "down."

   Since you are lying in semisupine, down is toward your pelvis not the floor. Do not drop your eyes. Summon an awareness of the space this is toward your pelvis and, in semisupine, toward your feet. As you practice thinking this direction, and each of the other spatial directions to follow, continue to keep in mind the general instructions in steps one and two above.

4. Shift back and forth: think *up*, then think *down*, then think *up*. Give each directional thought sufficient time to become clear in your awareness, and then change.

   What do you notice? Is it easier to think up or down? How do you feel throughout the whole of yourself as you think up, and then as you think down? Do they produce different effects in you?

5. Summon in your mind an awareness of the spatial direction that is "wide." This is like expanding out your ears—to the right and to the left simultaneously.

   Once you have a sense of the wide direction, allow this thought of sideward expansion to extend out beyond your physical self. Also, remember to keep seeing out in front of you. Be sure that you are thinking wide in both directions—to the right and left equally—and that you are not focusing downward into your body to find a *feeling* of wide.

6. Summon in your mind an awareness of the spatial direction that is "forward." This is a sense of expansion toward the front of your face, toward the ceiling as you are lying down.

   As you think forward you may become aware of a change in how your eyes focus. You may also become more aware of the space between objects.

7. Summon in your mind an awareness of the spatial direction that is "back." This is the direction behind you, toward the floor.

   Do not drop your eyes as you think back. Allow your imagination to conceive of the direction toward the space that is behind you.

8. Shift back and forth: think *forward*, then think *back*, then think *forward* again. Give each directional thought some time and then change direction.

   What do you notice? Which direction is easier for you to think? Do these directions affect you differently? Allow each spatial thought to spread throughout the whole of you.

Putting Directions Together

1. Think in the directions *up* and *down* simultaneously.

2. Think in the directions *wide* to the right and left simultaneously.

3. Think in the directions *forward* and *back* simultaneously.

4. In this step you will put these three dimensions together. Think in the directions *up-down*, then sustain this spatial thought in your mind as you add the thought *wide*, and then sustain these directions—*up-down* and *wide*—as you add the thought *forward-back*.

   By combining these directions, you are conceiving of space in three dimensions simultaneously. You are no longer visualizing in your mind a piece of paper expanding into a box. You are just thinking of space in all directions.

Putting these directions together is like juggling. You begin with one ball—the thought of up-down. You keep that ball going while you add a second—wide. Then you keep both up-down and wide without losing them as you add forward-back. You will probably drop one or two balls before you master juggling all three. If you lose a direction start from the beginning again, reestablishing them in their sequence. Each time you lose a spatial direction, you are presented an opportunity. Not only are you learning to think spatially, you are learning to recognize when you stop thinking spatially and to practice renewing this thinking.

Note: Throughout the remainder of these self-experiments, for brevity I will shorten the phrase "up-down, wide, and forward-back" to simply "up, wide, and forward."

5. Think in the direction that is the opposite of up-down. This is the direction that is *toward your center*, coming together from above and below. Then sustain this thought as you think *narrow*. This is the direction that is toward your midline, coming together from both sides of you. Sustain these as you think in the direction that is *inward*, coming together from forward and back toward your middle.

You are now thinking the opposite way from what you were thinking in step four. What do you notice? What has happened to your vision and your awareness of the room around you? What has happened to your breathing? How do you feel? What do you notice about your state of mind?

Note: Throughout the remainder of these self-experiments, for brevity I will shorten these instructions to refer to this simply as "down, narrow, and back."

6. Practice contrasting these thoughts: think in the directions *up*, *wide*, and *forward* for several minutes. Then think, *down*, *narrow*, and *back* for several minutes. Then change again.

How do these experiences compare? Does your breathing change? Is your mood affected? By shifting back and forth, most people experience a powerful sense of the difference. Thinking up, wide, and forward produces a sense of expansion, openness, and release. Thinking down, narrow, and back produces heaviness, tension, and even depression.

7. Think *up*, *wide*, and *forward*.

As you think, *up, wide, and forward,* summon the meaning of these words in yourself, and then let the words fall away as you sustain your awareness of three-dimensional space—all together and all at once—without any words at all.

Although you are summoning an awareness of the meaning of these words in your mind, also allow your thoughts of these spatial directions *to affect you physically.* Let them become embodied within you. They are not just mental abstractions; the words remind you to let yourself expand, three-dimensionally, throughout the whole of yourself.

Turning Your Head

1. Lie in semisupine as you think of quieting your voices. Rise up to your attic. Think, *up*, *wide*, and *forward*. Sustain your three-dimensional awareness as you turn your head *slowly* to the right. If you lose any of the directions, stop moving. Think, *up, wide, and forward* and begin again. When your head has turned as far as it can easily go (do not force this movement or rush), repeat this as you change direction, turning to the left.

In this experiment you are sustaining your directional thinking as you do a simple movement. It is also a test of the clarity of your directing. *It is important to understand that thinking three-dimensionally is in reference to—and moves with—your head, not your body or the space around you.* This means that as you turn your head to the right, your thought of "wide" is of a direction out both your ears—wide is not aligned with the position of your shoulders. And the forward-back thought is a direction of expansion in front of your face and out the back of your head—they are not aligned with the position of your torso.

Pay close attention to the moment that you change direction as you are turning your head. What happens to your spatial thinking? Do you think in the direction of the movement (right or left), rather than sustaining the directions? (As an alternative, remember to use the phrase, "up-down, wide, and forward–back.")

2. Expand on this experiment by practicing your spatial thinking in different activities: Sit in a chair, seeing out in front of you as you quiet your voices and rise up to your attic. Then *think*, *up*, *wide* and *forward*. Sustain this for several minutes and then continue as you stand up. Try thinking spatially as you walk, as you drive the car, as you read, or as you work at your computer. Have fun experimenting.

Forward and Up

1. Lie in semisupine. Quiet your voices. Rise up to your attic. Think in the direction *forward and up*. This direction is toward your hairline on your forehead. It is a diagonal, which is a combination of two spatial directions: up and forward. If you find it difficult to think in this direction, first think *up*, and then aim your up slightly *forward*.

   The forward and up direction that you want is a shallow diagonal, just slightly forward from the up direction that is toward the top of your head.

   Pay attention to the area of contact of your head on the books as you lie in semisupine. If the contact shifts lower, instead of thinking the direction, you are trying to do the direction in your muscles by tucking your chin back and tilting your head forward. If the contact shifts higher, you are trying to do the direction by pulling your head back.

2. Experiment by changing the angle of forward and up. First try thinking more *forward*. Then think more *upward*.

   Do you notice any changes in yourself as you change the angle of your forward and up?

3. Sit in a chair. Think, *forward and up*. Experiment with the angle of this direction. The importance of this direction should become clearer when you are upright.

4. While sitting, put your directing skills together: Think, *up*, *wide*, and *forward*. Establish your sense of three-dimensional space within you and around you. Let this affect the whole of yourself. Then continue thinking spatially as you aim your thought in the direction, *forward and up*.

▶ **DISCUSSION**

Thus far you have been practicing what I call the first two elements of the skill that Alexander teachers term *directing*. The first element, thinking *up, wide, and forward* is activating your mind's capacity to *conceive of three-dimensional space*. The second, *forward and up*, is activating your mind's capacity to *conceive of a specific direction within space*. Many people experience a wide array of benefits simply from thinking up, wide, and forward. Adding the direction forward and up further enhances your psychophysical coordination.

Thinking Names of Body Parts

1. Lie in semisupine. Quiet your voices and rise up to your attic. Think *up*, *wide*, and *forward* and then add the thought, *forward and up*. As you sustain your spatial thinking and this direction, say the names of different body parts to yourself: Neck. Knee. Stomach. Lower back. Pause after each one to notice how you respond.

   Does your attention shift down to the body part as you name it? Do you lose your spatial thinking or your direction forward and up as your mind tries to zero in on the body part you have just named? These words are stimuli that distract you from your directional thinking. They cause you to shift your attention down to your body and to feeling your body, rather than thinking of space.

▶ **DISCUSSION**

If you have already had Alexander lessons, you have probably noticed that what you have been practicing thus far is different from "saying the directions" as this is usually taught. My experience has convinced me that students learn to direct more quickly and effectively when they begin by practicing these three skills: spatial thinking; thinking in a specific spatial direction, particularly "forward and up"; and sustaining these as they practice thinking the names of parts of the body to learn not to focus on feeling as they direct.

There is another difference in my approach. Some teachers instruct their students to begin directing with the phrase "let the neck be free." I do not include this as a part of the directing instructions because it is not a spatial direction. It is a reminder to inhibit *before* you direct. In this respect it is important, since it is always a good idea to remind yourself to inhibit before you direct, and especially to inhibit tension in the neck. (I prefer using the phrase "I am not tensing my neck," which is a clearer inhibitory command.) In either case, beginning by thinking of not tensing in the neck is always a good idea so that the head is allowed to be mobile on top of the spine, and the neck is in a better alignment with the entire spine, as we discussed in chapter 18. Also, if you do not inhibit before you start to direct, *it is easy to forget that the directions are not instructions for fixing something that is wrong in your body by tensing your muscles, but for thinking of space.*

Now that you have practiced the three skills of thinking spatially, you are ready to learn to direct using Alexander's instructions and to discover how this adds another essential element to your skill.

Alexander's Directions

1. Lie in semisupine. Quiet your voices and rise up to your attic. Think to yourself, *I want to* not *tighten my neck.*

2. Think, *up, wide,* and *forward.*

3. Think, *I want to let my head be forward and up.*

   As you say these words, summon the meaning of the word "head" in your mind, *but do not try to do anything to your head with your muscles.* Next summon in your mind the thought of the direction "forward and up," *but do not try to do anything to make your head move in this direction.* Repeat this phrase, combining these two thoughts simultaneously in your mind: the meaning of the word head, and the direction forward and up. Repeat this a number of times: I want to let my head be forward and up.

4. Think, *I want to let my back lengthen up and widen.*

Conceive of the meaning of the word "back" without overfocusing on your back and trying to feel it or doing something with your muscles. Think the directions "up" (toward your head) and "wide" (expanding out your ears, right and left). Repeat this phrase a number of times: *I want to let my back lengthen up and widen.*

5. Think, *I want to let my knees release forward.*

This instruction can be difficult to understand. It does not mean to bend your knees. If you are standing, your knees should be straight (but not locked). This is an instruction for the whole of your legs. It means that the muscles of your thighs and lower legs should lengthen, so that the joints of your legs are available to bend when you move. Practice this phrase a number of times: *I want to let my knees release forward.*

6. Combine these phrases in sequence—*I want to not tighten my neck; I want to let my head be forward and up; I want to let my back lengthen up and widen; I want to let my knees release forward.*

Repeat this to yourself for about ten minutes until you can think these phrases in their sequence with ease. Remember to think of the meaning of the noun in each phrase, and then to think in the spatial direction toward which part of your body is being aimed: head, forward and up; back, lengthening up and widening; and knees, forward.

As each spatial direction in the series is established, you do not have to continue saying the words. The words are not the actual directional thought; they are the cue. They remind you to turn on a conscious directional awareness in your mind.

You want to sustain this awareness of each specific spatial direction in your mind as you add each succeeding direction. In time, thinking these phrases becomes like turning a key in the car's ignition. It initiates a type of thinking that triggers expansion—the expansion of your whole body, all its moveable parts in opposition, lengthening up, out, and away from each other.

7. **Additional Directions:** Sometimes Alexander used specific directions for the arms and hands: "to lengthen away from the shoulders and wrists toward the elbows," and "to lengthen the fingers away from the hands." Today many teachers have also expanded on these to include a direction for the feet, especially "to let the heels release down toward the ground."

▶ DISCUSSION

Keep in mind that Alexander's directions are not instructions for moving parts of your body correctly. They are not like the specific instructions that a coach or music teacher might give you to put your hands, arms, or legs in a certain position, or to move in a specific way. Thinking the directions is a cognitive skill that enlivens your mind's power to think three-dimensionally, and to think in specific spatial directions.

As you practice directing, it may be helpful to refer to Illustration 3-3. This shows the relative positions of the centers of gravity of your head, torso, and legs. We might say that Alexander's directions help you to think of each of these centers of weight moving away from each other in space to help you maintain the subtle and delicate counterbalance of all the parts of yourself. This counterbalance is the essential element of your bipedal design. If all your centers of weight are allowed to move away from one another, all your muscles lengthen slightly, which increases their tonus and strength. As a result, your muscles support you upright with length, expansion, and a minimum of effort rather than with tightening, shortening, and compression.

As you practice thinking the directions, you might experience a different sense of yourself. Students have varied reactions to directing. They sometimes describe themselves as feeling less attached to their body. Or they describe themselves as having a sense that they are not paying enough attention to specific parts of themselves, or that they are not trying hard enough to make their body move in the right way. Sometimes students describe themselves as not feeling as much. If you experience any of these, do not worry. These are all signs of increasing skill.

F MOVING WITH INHIBITION AND DIRECTION

Learning is the evolution of the mind.
—ALISON CROCKER

Now that you have learned to inhibit and direct, you are ready to put these skills to greater use. In this section you will return to bending a leg as you inhibit, this time by adding directing. In the process you will learn more about your psychophysical habits and beliefs. You will also practice using your new skills while doing simple movements, as you are upright. Remember to be patient, to allow yourself lots of time, and to enjoy the process of self-discovery.

Bending Your Leg

1. Lie in semisupine with one leg straight and the other leg bent. Begin by quieting your voices and shifting your attention upward as you think, *I am not moving my leg*, for several minutes.

2. Add to this your spatial thinking *up*, *wide*, and *forward* as you continue to remind yourself that you are not moving your leg.

   Continue seeing out in front of yourself as you repeat these words and summon their meaning within you. Establish in your mind a sense of three-dimensional space.

3. Continue to inhibit and direct thinking, *I am not moving my leg*, and thinking, *up*, *wide*, and *forward*. Then add the specific direction, *forward and up*. Sustain this as you wait and allow your *helper* to bend your leg.

   Once you begin to move your leg, notice if you stop directing and shift back to feeling.

   Do not be disappointed if you are unable to direct while moving. It is common to regress when you increase the difficulty of the task. In time you will be able to sustain your directional thinking while your helper moves you. When this happens, you will notice that the leg moves with even less effort than before. You will also have more awareness of the whole of yourself and the space around you as you move.

4. Use Alexander's directions: Think, *I am not moving my leg*, then think, *My neck is not tightening as I let my head release forward and up. My back is lengthening up and widening, and my knees are releasing forward.* Wait and allow your helper to move your leg as you sustain your inhibiting and directing.

Remember to think the meaning of the nouns—the names of your body parts (head, back, legs)—without trying to feel them or fix them. Think in spatial directions as you say these words to yourself. What do you discover?

Moving Forward and Back

1. Sit on the front of a chair that has a firm, level seat. Place your feet flat on the floor so that your heels are resting on the ground. Rest your hands on your thighs. As you are sitting but not moving, quiet your voices. Rise up to your attic. Think, *I am not sitting,* and allow your words, especially the word "not" to have meaning in your mind. Then direct: *I want to let my head release forward and up, my back to lengthen up and widen, my knees to release forward.*

Take time to think these instructions in their sequence, over and over. Do not worry if you are doing it right, or whether it is working. Do not be drawn downward to overfocus on feelings in your body. Simply sit as you inhibit—thinking of not sitting, and direct.

Next, you will experiment with a small movement as you continue inhibiting and directing. You will move your torso forward a few inches by bending forward from your hip joints. (You want your whole back to remain lengthening as you move rather than bending at your waist or curving forward in your chest.) Then you will swing back on your hip joints to return to the sitting position, again without bending in the waist or upper back. Try this small pivoting motion a few times to get a sense of it before you begin.

2. Rise up to your attic and think, *I am not sitting*. Continue this for several minutes. Then think, *I am* not *moving*. Then think spatially: *up, wide,* and *forward,* and add, *forward and up.* Once you have a sense of three-dimensional expansion in your mind, and of the specific direction forward and up, think of what you intend to do (lean forward) but do not *decide* to do it. Clarify in your mind your intention to move without deciding to move, which as you have learned will trigger your habitual muscle reaction. Inhibit and direct as you wait to let your helper do the movement.

3. After you have pivoted forward a few inches, stop moving and remain where you are. Renew your inhibiting and directing, and then move a few more inches forward. Then stop, inhibit and direct, and move forward again, and then stop again.

   Do you notice that when your torso is forward—away from vertical up—it is harder to sustain your inhibiting and directing? As we discussed in chapter 18, most of us have become habituated to the vertical. Once we leave this habitual orientation (the feeling of being upright and perpendicular to the ground) our brain becomes flooded with unfamiliar sensory inputs. When this happens, it becomes more difficult to direct. Do not be discouraged. Just stop wherever you are and take time to renew your thinking.

4. Repeat steps two and three as you move your torso back in space to return to the upright sitting position. Be sure to take time to stop and renew your inhibiting and directing whenever necessary, and then continue.

   As you practice, notice if your thinking tends to shift down or backward, or if your attention focuses itself on a part of your body, or if your mind wanders. When you notice something of this sort, stop what you are doing, return to your attic, inhibit, think the directions, and start again. As you succeed in sustaining your inhibiting and directing as you move, notice if your pattern of coordination changes also.

5. Now you will move in a slightly more challenging way. Begin sitting. Inhibit: think of not sitting, and not moving. Direct. Then move your

torso backward in space so that you are leaning slightly back from the vertical. Then stop and renew your inhibiting and directing, and then move a little farther back, and so on. Then return your body to the vertical sitting position in the same way.

As you try this, give particular attention to your forward direction. The thought of forward often disappears as we move back in space. In the blink of an eye, your mind will shift its attention to the feeling of moving back. When this happens, stop moving, inhibit, direct, and then move again. In this experiment you are learning to sustain your directing, regardless of where you are moving your torso in space.

Try the same movements as you think Alexander's directions:

6. Begin by thinking, *I am* not *going to move.* Then think, *I want to let my head release forward and up, to let my back lengthen up and widen, to let my knees release forward.* Repeat this phrase over to yourself for several minutes. Think the first direction, then the next and the next, one after the other and all together as you start to move, pivoting your torso forward and backward in the chair.

Remember not to focus on the sensations of your body as you move. You are not trying to feel what is happening, or judging this feeling, or deciding how to do the movement correctly. You do not want to use your mind to focus on feeling where you are moving in space. You are directing to coordinate your body headward and to orient yourself relative to the ground. Use your mind to direct—aiming and coordinating yourself in space as a three-dimensional being in motion.

▶ DISCUSSION

You may notice subtle changes in the clarity and accuracy of your directing. Sometimes it will seem easy, at other times more difficult. By practicing, you will get better, but this does not mean that your progress will proceed in a straight line, or that your thinking will become perfect and you will not have to bother with it anymore. Subtle variations in your state of being from day to day and even moment to moment will affect your skill at each moment.

Remember to keep your eyes open and seeing out in front of you as you move. Do not let your eyes drop down and focus inward. This usually means your directing is not all it might be.

As you practice, you will become more skilled at noticing in your peripheral awareness the subtle sensory clues that indicate you are coordinating yourself more efficiently. You can note this with interest, but remember that your chief goal is to sustain your inhibiting and directing, not to focus on the sensations of the movement—bad or good. It is the quality of your thought that you want to perceive with accuracy, not the correctness or rightness of the movement of your body.

Standing and Sitting

1. Begin from a sitting position. Take time to inhibit, thinking, *I am* not *sitting,* and then think, *I am* not *standing up.* Continue to inhibit as you direct your head to release forward and up, your back to lengthen up and widen, and your knees to release forward. Sustain this thinking for a period of time. Continue inhibiting and directing and wait for your helper to stand you. (Alternatively, you can use just the directions *up, wide,* and *forward,* and *forward and up.*)

   If you notice your mind shift to thinking about how you will stand, or when you will stand, or how it feels to begin to stand, you know that you have stopped inhibiting.

2. Once you are standing, repeat the same process. Think, *I am* not *standing,* and then, *I am* not *sitting down.* Clarify your intention to sit without deciding to sit. Think your directions. Wait for your helper to begin the movement rather than deciding to sit.

   What do you discover?

TOUCH
OUR FORGOTTEN SENSE

Touching the Heart

The most beautiful thing we can experience is the mysterious.
It is the source of all true art and science.

—ALBERT EINSTEIN

SAM

Today I AM seeing Sam, a student who has been taking lessons with me for several years. Sam is in his sixties, tall, with large hands and feet, a tumbled mess of white hair, and warm, round eyes. He is bright, personable, and a bit shy. He loves the lessons, asks thoughtful questions, reports on his insights, and enjoys the process of change. Summer vacation and a business trip have meant a four-month hiatus in his lessons. I am looking forward to seeing him and hearing his news.

When Sam walks in my door I am taken aback. His smile is genuine but muted. His eyes do not engage with mine; his voice is muffled. He walks slowly and seems more bent over than usual. Sam knows how to inhibit and direct, but today I wonder if he has forgotten all he has learned. I find myself feeling concerned and probe gently to discern any problems, but he does not mention anything. It is possible I am misreading the cues, I tell myself.

Since Sam looks tired, I suggest that he lie on the table. I begin by lifting and turning his head, feeling his neck's mobility. As I do this, I remind him to think of rising up to his attic to quiet his inner chatter, then to think of not tensing his neck. Next I place my hands on his shoulders. They feel tense and stiff. Usually the combination of Sam's inhibition and my hands-on contact produces a softening release in his muscles. Today, nothing changes. I take my hands off his shoulders and continue working, gently supporting each arm in its turn, reminding him to think of not tightening, then to think of directing his head forward and up, his torso to lengthen up and widen, his knees to free forward. I move on to his legs, supporting each leg as I ask him to think of not moving and to allow me to move his leg for him.

I observe Sam closely as I give him verbal instructions, and use my hands to feel what he is doing within himself. My hands scan for information that cannot be seen. They suggest that muscular release is possible, that joints can bend freely. At the same time, they feel the answering response from the student. Often I think of my hands like the metal detectors people use at the beach, sweeping over the sand, beeping their signal of hidden treasure.

Noticing that Sam's ribcage is barely moving, which means he is not breathing well, I place a hand lightly on his sternum (the long flat bone at the front of the chest). Then I ask him to think of not holding his ribs. A moment later, I feel a sudden, powerful pressure against my chest, as if a fifty-pound weight is pressing on my sternum. It is not a subtle sensation, and I have never experienced anything like it before. Trying not to show my distress, I remove my hand and stand beside the table, taking time to collect myself.

What does this mean?

After a moment the sensation passes and I feel better. Not wanting to interrupt the lesson, I decide to carry on. A few minutes later, since I am feeling fine again, I notice that Sam is still not breathing well. I place my hand on his sternum again. The same powerful feeling of compression arises in my chest.

What is wrong? Am I having a heart attack?

I remove my hand again. Soon I am feeling better. Then it crosses my mind that what I am feeling might have something to do with Sam rather than me. Deciding to experiment, I put my hand on his chest a third time. Again I experience the same heavy, pressing sensation. I look at Sam. He does not seem to notice me, or to be wondering what I am doing. He looks subdued, inwardly focused. I take my hand off and the sensation evaporates.

I am more than a little perplexed by these events, but we both seem to be functioning well enough so I decide to continue the lesson. I help Sam off the table and we work standing and sitting in the chair, and then walking. The lesson over, Sam departs with a meager smile. He does not appear to have changed at all, and I find myself worrying if there is something seriously wrong with him.

A few days later Sam's wife, Joanne, calls me. She is also a student, and we have a comfortable, trusting relationship. She says she has called to tell me that Sam has been suffering from a severe depression, which began a few months before. She adds that he will not be coming for lessons for a while, as he is seeing a doctor and having tests to determine its cause. She promises to call when they know more.

I thank her for calling, express my concern, and say good-bye. I choose not to tell her about my experience during Sam's lesson, but as I think back, the mystery clears. My hunch was correct. The pressure I felt as I placed my hand on Sam's chest was not my own. Somehow I was feeling, I guess you could say, the weight of his depression. But how I was able to feel this in myself I cannot begin to rationally explain.

WHAT IS IT ABOUT TOUCH?

Years ago in high school I peered through a microscope in biology class and watched, transfixed, as a single-celled paramecium propelled itself with its cilia foot across my slide. Then the creature bumped into another of its kind, paused, flicked its tail, and moved away. Paramecia bumping into each other cannot be said to recognize one another or to feel the experience, but this simple contact marks a beginning: Where else to launch our evolution as sensate beings than with the capacity to register our body's property line? Touch is our first and perhaps most essential sense. It is through the sensory system of touch that we learn about and experience the world outside ourselves.

Yet this simple account has some flaws. When we touch something, we are not exactly learning about external objects. Usually we say that when we hold a rock, for example, we learn that rocks are cold, rough, and hard. To be more precise, we should say that holding a rock allows us to experience the sensations of coldness, roughness, and hardness *within ourselves*. In other words, we can only perceive the rock as having the qualities that the sensory receptors in our fingers are capable of discerning.

In addition, many of the sensations we experience from our skin are triggered without touching anything at all. (If you have had a case of poison ivy, you know that a maddening itch can arise from your skin without any contact.)

Wouldn't it be more logical then to rename our sense of touch our *sense of skin*?

Or perhaps it would be more consistent to include the sense of touch within our sixth sense, the sense of bodily sensation, since touching causes us to feel and know something within ourselves. Or these two sensory systems could be combined and given an entirely new classification. What if we were to name all the sensory experiences of the body our *sense of feeling*?

Whatever we name this sensory system and however we categorize it, let us begin our discussion of touch with the material side of the story.

Traversing many evolutionary miles—from the single-celled organism's cell wall to the complex sensory capacities of the human hand—the skin covering our body is our largest, heaviest organ. This outermost layer of ourselves contains a huge number and variety of specialized sensory receptors and nerve endings. There are specific types of sensory receptors that are sensitive to hot, cold, pressure, the absence of pressure, pain, and much more. When these receptors are stimulated, singly or in combination, they yield an astonishing complexity of feelings: soft, hard, slippery, wet, cold, hot, smooth, bumpy, fuzzy, pressure, slight pain, medium pain, stabbing pain, dull pain, tickling, sexual arousal, buzzing, itching, numbness, etc.

According to scientists at M.I.T. delving into the mechanisms of touch, the skin on our fingertips is especially sensitive.[1] Each fingertip contains at least two thousand specialized sensory receptors enabling us to feel a dot just three microns high. (A human hair's diameter is 50 to 100 microns.) If we feel a texture rather than a dot, we can detect roughness just 75 nanometers high—about one one-hundredth of a micron.

But touch is not simply the province of our fingertips and hands; it abides in the entire wraparound envelope that is our skin, our outer frontier. Once the skin's myriad sensory receptors are stimulated, wherever they are located, they send their electrical signals onward via sensory nerves. Touch leads us, as do all our senses, to the brain, where we arrive at the perceptual realm. The impulses from our skin are summed up and the raw grit of data transformed. It is the mind that conjures its sensory picture. First, it locates the origin of the message. (*Is that sensation in my left hand?*) It decides what the message means. (*Is that pain?*) Then it makes a judgment. (*Not good.*) Finally it selects a course of action. (*It will feel better if I rub it.*) Much of this incoming data does not reach our conscious awareness. The brain selects which stimuli will arrive on the desktop of our awareness for further consideration, and which will not.

These touch images are a terrifically complex creation, which are in turn shaped by the self that our lifetime of touching has helped to create. Memories, beliefs, learning, emotions, even our level of alertness at a given moment affect our tactile perceptions. It is harder to relax in the dentist's chair when you know that you might feel pain, and your anxiety makes your perception of the pain increase. You are not quite as ticklish when you are almost asleep and deeply relaxed. If you are sitting at your desk, absorbed in paying the bills as someone walks quietly into the room and touches you gently on the shoulder, you may jump an inch off the chair in sudden (and unnecessary) alarm.

Touch, like all our senses, brings us a way of knowing. With or without our conscious awareness, it generates meaning. When we touch, we are altered. The meaning that we give to the object that we touch also affects the way that we touch, and our perception of how this feels. Consider the difference in how you feel as you hold a plastic plate as compared with how you feel as you hold a valuable plate made of fine bone china. Your belief about the relative value and fragility of these objects gives your experience a distinctly different character.[2]

When we speak of touch, we often fail to distinguish between touching an inanimate object and touching an animate one, especially touching our own kind. Do you feel the same when you hold a fake rose as opposed to a real one? Does the soft, fuzzy, stuffed dog feel the same as the genuine thing? When we touch another living being, there is shared experience. Our touch conveys something to the other at the same moment that it brings something to us. Touch between creatures is more than mere contact. It is a forerunner to language, an act of communication between sentient beings. The messages that are conveyed can be vital, and touch becomes far more than the exchange of stimuli. The experience of touch and the act of touching are essential to who we are, how we behave, and even to our existence.

Consider a few examples of communication through touch in the animal kingdom: ants crossing the kitchen floor en route to the honey jar, stopping to greet their oncoming brethren with a touch of antennae; puppies playing, tumbling head over feet and all over each other; chimps sitting for hours, languorously grooming one another; bees dancing in the hive, bumping and tapping, bodies and wings touching in meaningful discussion—the petunias are that way!

As for yourself, have you ever been touched by a bored lover? Does it feel the same as when you are touched by someone who deeply feels their love for you, someone who in the moment of touching is engaged in the expression of this love? To the objective eye, the touch may appear the same. It may bear the same pressure. It may be placed identically on the body and move in the same direction. But the meaning expressed and experienced by you is different. There is something more that is conveyed beyond contact and pressure.

Studies conducted in the 1960s showed that young monkeys raised without any touch were significantly impaired psychologically, as compared with their normally raised peers. Monkeys that were raised alone but had a surrogate mother made of wire and terry cloth to touch and hold were more normal.

The mothers of many species lick their young after birth, covering their entire bodies. This is more than cleansing behavior. The sensory stimulation the newborn receives through its skin is essential for normal brain development. Premature human babies gain more weight, and have better survival rates, when they are held by caregivers and massaged than when they are relegated to the seemingly optimal conditions of the incubator. Skin-to-skin contact diminishes our stress hormone levels and heightens our immune response. Receiving a foot rub when you are tense and anxious provides more than pleasant sensation. Within minutes you feel calmer; the clouds hovering over your brain have dissipated. Sensory stimulation to your foot alters your mind's biochemistry, transforming your mood. Scientists have confirmed what we all know in our hearts: lonely people, and especially the elderly, are happier and live longer when they have an animal to hold. Touch between living beings is a language that conveys something beyond stimulation and sensation; it gives us something we need, physiologically, body and soul.

I remember holding my six-month-old son in my arms and feeling his small hands touching my face. His touch had a remarkable quality. His palms were spread wide and his fingers extended. Ten fingers and two palms made definite contact on my cheeks, yet they felt like billowing clouds. It seemed there were no hard bones or hardening muscles within them. He was not using his hands to manipulate or hold me, but to feel and know me. His hands behaved like the exploratory wanderings of an animal examining its world, not the grasping instruments of the human adult. It was a vivid moment of shared expression.

Could we venture to say that without touch not only could we not express love, we could not learn to know its meaning? The neurons of the hand and the skin are connected to the brain and vice versa. Through touch we speak our minds and hearts to the perimeter of ourselves and in contact pass this along, while simultaneously absorbing something from the one we are touching. How is it that this is conveyed and received? We have left behind the material level of sensory receptors and firing neurons. The expression of the self through touch is an ineffable mystery.

It is perplexing that this capacity we all share is so widely ignored. We might expect that we would want to better understand it and make the fullest use of this capacity. The sad fact is there is little regard for touch in our culture. Touching is taboo. It is shunted away, relegated to the provinces of sexuality and maternity, and then dismissed. It seems to be too discomfiting.

Let me offer a few more examples. A friend tells me about a personally painful experience. I reach out and put a hand on his shoulder to offer a physical expression of concern and sympathy. Rather than receive my touch, he recoils with a jolt as if he had bumped into a hot stove. How does the touch of a friend's hand become an alarming event? I have often thought that children from abusive homes who are violent and aggressive ought to receive daily foot rubs and massages. Since touch can alter the state of our brain, what better more direct route for easing the disturbance and static of a troubled mind?

When I am teaching I frequently ask students to put a hand on me. If I have been talking about rib mobility, for example, I might ask a student to place her hands on the sides of my rib cage to feel how ribs move in respiration. As she does this, her fingers curl and grip, pressing uncomfortably hard.

"No," I instruct, "let go of your muscles. Place your fingers lightly. Tensing muscles doesn't help you to feel. Just make contact. Allow your hands to open. You'll be able to feel more." Even after this instruction, my student is usually unable to do as I suggest. The prospect of touching makes her anxious, or perhaps she believes that to touch means she must do something. As a result she tenses her muscles, and this contraction gives me the felt experience of her anxiety.

Teachers in public schools are not permitted to touch students. I know an Alexander teacher who was offered a job at a performing arts high school, only to be told that the course had to be cancelled due to the hands-on aspect of the instruction. Our culture prizes the fruits of our other senses: the visual arts, music, fine cuisine. But the education and training of our sense of touch is not permitted. Touch isn't valued; it is considered dangerous. The anthropologist John Napier, known for his study and analysis of the human hand, epitomizes this tone of compartmentalization: "The movement of the thumb underlies all the skilled procedures of which the hand, is capable."[3] In short, the masterpiece of the human hand is viewed as the locus of our doing, achieving, conquering selves. The gentle act of giving, receiving, and educating through touch is barely known.

What has become of the simple act of touching our own kind from childhood to adulthood? Why do we not value the young child's extending, open, seeking-to-know hands? How is it that we come to view our hands only as tools? Our appreciation for touch lies lost like a sunken ship on the seabed.

A notable exception is the skilled Alexander teacher. A product myself of the cultural norm when I scheduled my first appointment for a lesson, I had no idea what was in store for me. I still recall the extraordinary quality of my teacher's touch, and the physical and mental changes her hands produced. She began the lesson by asking me to lie on my back with my knees bent. A short while later she was standing beside me, gently lifting and supporting my arm. I became aware of my muscles lengthening. A moment later my muscles seemed to reach their limit for stretch. At what seemed to be the same moment, she stopped moving my arm and held it. After another moment, the muscles of my arm and shoulder released again. She moved my arm a little more. This stopping and starting process was repeated several times. A few minutes later I was certain she had lengthened my arm by at least four inches.

"How did she do that?" I wondered later as I described it to a friend. "She moved me in a way I've never experienced. My muscles released and my arm lengthened, but she didn't DO anything. She didn't pull or push on my muscles. She just held my arm and my muscles released. It seemed as if her hands talked to my body and my body talked to her. How did she do that?" I repeated, mystified.

The feeling was marvelous, but it was the conversation that took place between my body and my teacher's hands that really caught my attention. Her hands seemed to know what my body was doing better than I did. They spoke something to which my muscles responded, without my conscious mind knowing exactly what that was or deciding what should happen and then doing it.

Later, as an Alexander teacher-in-training, I learned that this marvelous skill was the result of specialized and intensive study. The more I experienced the nuances of this skill, the more astonished I became. Today, more than thirty years later, my understanding of the art and use of the hands has not reached its limit. Like the professional musician, whose mastery of his instrument is never complete despite a lifetime of study, so it is for the Alexander teacher's skilled touch.

The teacher's hands serve two functions simultaneously. First, they convey an experience to the student. This is not a matter of using the hands to massage muscles or manipulate the body. The student experiences a gentle contact that lightly supports, guides, energizes, expands, and informs how the student moves. Second, the teacher's hands feel what the student does to his body: how he moves and reacts, and how he responds to the teacher's instruction. This information can only be gained through touch. The teacher is able to feel what we would call the student's psychophysical pattern of response—how the student uses himself in that moment, mind and body. This knowledge enables the teacher to adjust the hands-on guidance and verbal instruction appropriately to the individual.

Sometimes a student asks me to explain what I am doing with my hands. Since words cannot capture it, I offer a brief demonstration. The student may be lying in semisupine as I place my palms lightly on his leg.

"Close your eyes," I instruct. "This is the first type of contact from my hands. Go ahead and let yourself focus on feeling my hands.

Now I am going to change something—not in my hands, specifically, but in my thinking." After a moment's pause I ask, "This is the second contact. Do you experience a difference?"

"Yes, but it's hard to describe. The first time your hands felt less alive. They felt warm and nice; the touch was okay; but nothing happened in me. In fact I felt a bit more closed in, compressed."

"And the second time?"

"It was different. You didn't do anything, but I felt freer. Your hands seemed more energized. They conveyed something to my muscles. I was breathing better and my muscles released."

"Good. We've demonstrated a fundamental principle of the Alexander Technique. What the teacher is doing, psychophysically, as she touches the student affects the hands-on contact. If I have my hands on you while I am tense and mentally distracted, my touch is not as clear or effective. If I am inhibiting and directing as I touch you, my hands will convey this. My own release and expansion encourages you to do the same. It doesn't guarantee that this will happen. I can't make you let go of your muscles if you don't want to, but if you don't interfere, my hands communicate my state of being to you. They invite you to change. So I must practice what I preach. I'm not standing here telling you what you should do and how you should do it. I am seeking to use myself well, and inviting you to do the same."

21

The Teacher's Hands

A light, tender, sensitive touch is worth a ton of brawn.
—PETER THOMSON

TONIGHT I AM addressing a group of teachers who attend my monthly postgraduate seminar. Their questions range from business details to anatomical fine points to pedagogy. They always present me with thoughtful questions, but some are harder to answer than others. These are the questions that, I must admit, I hope they do not ask. If pressed for a label I would call them questions about "mysterious phenomena." Tonight someone asks about the heart of the matter.

"How do you know what you're feeling with your hands?"

I catch my breath as my eyes drop to the floor. Uncertainty envelops me. It is not that I do not want to address this topic. Rather, I wonder if I can do it justice. Some experiences are so extraordinary that we long to share them with others, but talking only seems to trivialize them. Translated into the light of language, their truth becomes distorted. I put my hands on students every day, but can I explain how I know what this means? Do I risk creating more confusion by trying to explain what cannot be explained, or is some explanation—even an imperfect one—better than nothing?

After a moment I make my decision.

"All right, let's tackle this tonight. Here's what I suggest. I'll work on someone standing and sitting in the chair, and talk about what I am experiencing as I try to know what I'm feeling with my hands. Is that all right?" I see smiles and nodding heads.

"Anne, would you like to come up here?"

Anne smiles her assent and walks to the chair in the center of the room, turning to face the group. I stand next to her on her left. I place my right hand on her midback, my left hand on her lower ribs. As I do this, suddenly my mental focus blurs. Fear is rising within me like a thick cloud, threatening to blanket my mental faculties. Over the years I have learned what to do about this—I inhibit my reaction. I remind myself to go up to my attic as I tell myself not to pay attention to the feelings of anxiety and disorientation welling up within me. Soon they release their hold on my mind. Next an inner voice whispers, "You don't know what you're doing. You don't feel anything special, just a warm torso under your hands." It is the familiar voice of self-doubt. More fear. I disregard it as well, inhibit, and wait.

Then something shifts. It seems as if my hands become the metal prongs of an electric plug, extending into the socket. My palms spread; my fingers lengthen. My hands no longer barely touch the student but make broader contact. My ribs move readily as my eyes focus. Now it seems as if my student and I are connected—a two-way channel of communication opens between us. My mental clarity reemerges like a timid child, peering out from behind its mother's skirt. This is the moment I refer to as *getting plugged in*.

The teachers attending the seminar are familiar with my jargon. In passing I remark, "Okay, I'm plugged in to Anne. My hands are making contact. The point to emphasize is that I don't use muscular effort to achieve this contact. I place my hands on her, inhibit, and wait. This is crucial. I want to feel what is happening with my hands, but it doesn't happen the moment I touch her. It takes time for a sensory picture to come into view.

"Why is this exactly?" I ask. "We want to know what we are feeling with our hands. There are two components to this: *being able to feel the student*, and *understanding what the feeling means*. These are not the same. *The first step is to become able to feel; to do that, I must create the conditions in myself that allow me to receive sensory information.*

Essentially, the task is to clear the decks. If I am worried or fearful, my mind is wandering, or I am tense, I cannot receive sensory information from my hands as fully. The static of my emotions and muscle tension distorts the signal; or uses up the available sensory pathways; or maybe it occupies too much mental space, crowding out a simple clarity of perception.

"In any case, I begin by inhibiting. Gradually I become less distracted, mentally and physically. Then I gain a fuller hands-on contact and a sense of being plugged in to the student. What emerges in myself is what I like to call an **expanding field of awareness**. This is like climbing to the top of a mountain to get a better view: I can be aware of myself and my student simultaneously. This is the foundation on which everything else is built, so taking time for this to emerge is essential."

"When you say that you're inhibiting, can you say more about what you're thinking?"

"Sure. When I put my hands on the student, I am usually triggered into some level of fear reaction, even though this may be small. What's there to be afraid of? I couldn't say. In this case, I've known Anne for years. Is it performance anxiety? Maybe the student won't like me. But whenever you first put your hands on someone, it's jarring. It's like two bare wires touching and making sparks. So I go to my attic, quiet the chatter in my mind, and think, *I don't have to react,* or *I don't have to do anything,* or *I'm not putting my hands on anyone.* Then I wait. The static slowly subsides, my hands make better contact, and this state of expanding awareness emerges.

"There are some pitfalls that get in the way. For example, if we believe that we can only think one thing at a time, then when we put our hands on we create a split in our awareness—we focus on either the student or ourself. And if we believe it is our job to feel the student, we give all our attention to what we feel of the student in our hands, and we shut off our self-awareness.

"Let me demonstrate. With my hands on Anne, I'll tell myself to focus on feeling what's happening in her. What do you see?"

"You look pulled down in yourself."

"You look as though your attention is focused downward."

"You don't seem aware of what's going on around you."

"Yes. I'm doing all those things. Can everyone see that?" There is agreement around the room.

"Now I'll inhibit, and wait for my expanding awareness." After a moment I turn my head to look at the others. "Can you see a difference?"

"It's subtle, but you look more expanded and up."

"The expression on your face is different. You look calmer."

"Yes. What did I change? I stopped concentrating on feeling Anne with my hands. It is like tuning the dial on a radio to get better reception. By inhibiting, I create the conditions in myself that enable me to feel. Ironically, it's an erroneous belief about what it means to feel that interferes with being able to feel."

"Can you say more about what you mean by that?"

"Let's think about this neurologically. When you touch, sensory receptors are triggered in your skin, muscles, and joints. These receptors send signals that are processed in your brain. Then you say that you're feeling something in the student. But the feeling isn't really in the student, or in your hands. As you touch, what you feel comes to your awareness via sensory nerves that your brain receives and processes. What you're feeling is happening within you. It's an illusion to think you're feeling the other person. *You're feeling what touching the other person makes you feel in yourself.*

"This is a perplexing state of affairs. The good news is that you don't have to tune out yourself in order to tune in on the student. You can receive information from your hands while also receiving information about yourself. This is the state of expanding awareness that I am speaking of.

"It's also important to remember when you put your hands on that you have just one sensory system—and one brain—for receiving and processing information about two people. So things can get confusing. Your expanding awareness means that your mind is watching two television screens at once—you and the student. Sometimes these pictures overlap. It's as if they become superimposed, one on top of the other. Then it's difficult to see either picture, and easy to mistake parts of one for the other. Let me tell you a story to illustrate this.

"Years ago I gave a lesson to a student who had knee pain. One day as we finished, she said her pain was gone. After she left, I realized that I had pain in my knee. In fact, my pain was in the same place as my student's. I don't mean to say by this that she gave me her pain. Some people characterize this phenomenon in that way and it's a mistake. It gives a wrong impression, as though some noxious substance has been exchanged between student and teacher via the hands-on contact. But my mind was mistaking the sensory information about my student for information about me.

"This is key, because it's a source of burnout for teachers and caregivers. In our effort to empathize with the student and feel with our hands, we confuse the sensory impressions that come from the student with those that come from ourselves. To distinguish more clearly which is which, it's vital to maintain a sort of separation in your mind. You want to establish two screens of awareness—an expanding field of awareness that includes yourself and the student—but also keeps each screen distinct."

"How do you do that?"

"It boils down to inhibiting and directing. Inhibiting gives me the mental clarity to achieve this broader awareness. Directing helps me keep the two fields separate. As I direct, I am sending thoughts by me to me. I also receive the sensory feedback this generates. For example, if I have the thought to let my head go forward and up, I know it is I who is thinking and who is experiencing the sensory feedback this generates. It helps my mind make a distinction between sensory inputs. It's not foolproof, but it helps.

"Now let's talk about how I learn to understand the meaning of what I feel. It is possible to feel a great deal with your hands but not to know what it means. Learning to understand what you feel is a complex process that unfolds as you teach. Let me break this down into some discernible components.

"*The first step is to create contrasts that give you a means of comparison.* The easiest way to do this is through movement: You can move your hands to different places on the student, and you can move the student—in whole or in part.

"For example, I can put my hands on Anne's head and neck, then her ribs, then her shoulders. In this way my hands bring me a fuller awareness of the whole of her. I can also gather information by moving her. This doesn't have to be a large movement. Now I'm pivoting her slightly forward and backward from her ankles as she is standing. It is such a small movement that the student may not be aware of it. But as I move her, I feel her changing. I compare these changes and ask myself questions: Is she lighter than before or heavier? Is she lengthening upward or pulling down? Has she reacted, tensing as I move her, perhaps by pulling her head back and stiffening her neck? Or is she allowing me to move her without reacting? By noticing these before-and-after contrasts, I learn the meaning of what I'm feeling.

"But when you start to do something—either by moving your hands or by moving the student—there's another pitfall. Anybody know what that is?" I look around the room but no one speaks.

"Let's do what we did before. I'll move Anne in and out of the chair. Watch me and tell me what you see."

After a minute someone says, "Well, you look kind of down again. You've lost your up direction?"

"Right. What else do you notice?"

"Your thinking changed?"

"Yes. What happened to my thinking and my expanded field of awareness? Am I focused on Anne as I was before?"

"No, this time it looks like you're focused on yourself."

"That's right. This time instead of forgetting myself in an effort to feel Anne, I forgot about Anne while I focused on myself. When I began moving my arms, my attention shifted to the sensations in my body. My attention shifted to me. I stopped inhibiting and directing, and I forgot about Anne. Now I have to start at the beginning. I'll stop moving Anne for a moment and give myself time. This is better. I'm inhibiting and getting plugged in. My awareness is expanding. Now I'm directing."

"It really is amazing," Anne chimes in.

"What?" I ask.

"The quality of your hands really does change. You didn't move your hands or do anything to me just then, but I felt a distinct difference when you focused on me or on yourself, as opposed to now when you're inhibiting and directing. Before I felt imposed on and sort of pressed down, smaller. Now I feel as though you've given me space. I expand and lengthen upward. I'm breathing better. I even seem to get a better sense of you, the person behind the hands."

"Well, that says it nicely. This is what we want, right? We want to create the best possible psychophysical condition in ourselves and to sustain this as we use our hands, both to feel the student and to convey something to the student. It doesn't guarantee that something will change, but it creates an opportunity for something to change. Does that describe it accurately from your side, Anne?"

"Definitely."

"Returning to our topic of learning to know what we're feeling, I'm moving her and moving my hands to notice contrasts. Right now I'm feeling that Anne is light, not heavy; she's lengthening upward in her torso, not pulling down; her ribs are moving; she isn't collapsing as she exhales. I'm generating a picture in my mind that is fuller, more richly detailed.

"There's yet another pitfall, however. Once we're feeling more and understanding what we're feeling, we start to judge the student's misuse. Then we think about fixing it by doing something with our hands and worrying if we're doing this right, which creates anxiety. Just as we were getting going, we short-circuited the process. Do any of you find yourselves doing that?" I look at the group and see expressions of chagrin.

"But," someone asks, "what are you trying to feel if it isn't what the student is doing wrong? Don't you want to know whether the student is pulling her head back and down, or tightening in her back, and so on, and then use your hands to correct this? Isn't that the teacher's job?"

"You're asking important questions, but instead of answering them directly, I'm going to ask one in return. Since we want to learn to know what we're feeling with our hands, shouldn't we ask the question, *What is it that we want to know?* What are we using our hands to find out? Do I use my hands to know if she has rough skin, for example? No. Do I use my hands to find out what she is 'doing wrong,' as you've said? Well, sort of, but not for the reason you state. So let's talk about what I want to know and how I know it, and then about what I do with this information.

"I gather information from my hands on three levels. *First, my hands give me detailed information about the specific area that I'm touching.* We could call this the *musculoskeletal level.* I can put my hands on Anne's head and neck, for example, and feel if the muscles of her neck are hard or soft, if her head is easily mobile or stiffly resistant to movement. I can feel whether her head is tilted, rotated, or pulled down; or if her neck is overly curved or flattened; or if there's a narrowing constriction in her muscles.

"How do I know what I'm feeling at the musculoskeletal level? Knowledge of anatomy is very important. I can picture in my mind those neck vertebrae, how they interlock and the relative position of the bones, where the muscles insert and the nature of their action. This knowledge, combined with the information from my hands, gives me a lot of information about my student on a specific physical and mechanical level. It's tempting to focus my attention entirely on this because it's concrete. But my conception of what I'm trying to know is limited. If I focus only on anatomical details, I'll miss a lot of other vital information.

"*At the second level, my hands enable me to know something about how my student functions and behaves as a psychophysical whole.* My hands allow me to know about the student's connectedness: How her head is connected to her neck. How her head and neck are connected to her torso. How her torso is connected to her arms and legs. How this pattern of connection enhances or interferes with her headward coordination. I feel how her mind and body interact, connecting feeling and thinking, intention and action, unconscious habit and conscious awareness. I feel how my student responds with her whole self as she engages that self in activity.

"My hands bring me information about this whole person that I can't learn through any other means. I can't learn this from an anatomy book. Anatomy is the study of the parts of the body, not the study of the relationship among these parts in a living, functioning organism. Anatomy can never fully inform me about the gestalt that is my student. My hands feel what can't be seen, heard, or grasped intellectually through verbal description.

"At this level, my ability to know what I'm feeling comes primarily from my study and experience of my own use, and what this has taught me about mind-body connection. The textbook is myself. I don't mean to say that I must have the same habits of misuse as my student in order to understand hers. However, my study of the psychophysical mechanisms of misuse, especially of my head, neck, and back as they operate in me play a large part in my capacity to feel and understand this in the student.

"Now that I know something about my student's *disconnection*—her pattern of psychophysical misuse—how do I change it? Do I use my hands to fix her—to put each of her skewed body parts in their right places? Is it my responsibility to make her move correctly? Well, if my conception of her were of a physical object, moving and behaving along strictly mechanical and anatomical lines, this would be the thing to do. But my student isn't a body, and I'm not just working on a body. This is not bodywork. My student has thoughts, feelings, beliefs, and judgments. I must enter this arena as well. First, because my student's mind and body are a functional whole; and second, because it's the only way to make lasting change in her psychophysical habits of reaction.

"This brings me to the third level—*My hands enable me to know if my student is inhibiting and directing.* My hands are the best means for knowing this, since her inhibiting and directing thoughts are reflected outward onto the canvas of her physical self. It is my chief aim to teach my student how to think effectively, so that she can use these skills to change harmful and habitual behavior. My hands feel the release and lengthening that her inhibition allows in her muscles, the increased mobility in her joints, and the quiet calm this restores to her nervous system. My hands feel the dimensionality, lightness, headward coordination, and connectedness that emerge when she directs as I move her. My hands also enable me to give her tailor-made feedback to help her learn and then use these skills, and to better perceive how they enhance what she is doing.

"How do I feel inhibiting and directing in the student? Again, this is linked to myself. It comes from my experience and use of these skills in the present moment as I'm teaching. I can only feel my student's inhibiting and directing if I have learned how to inhibit and direct myself. The other main element, of course, is lots of practice.

"Let's return to Anne. I'll discuss what I'm feeling as I work on her, and try to show how these three levels of knowing through my hands come together as I'm teaching. I'll begin with something simple. I have my right hand under Anne's left elbow, and my left hand is holding her left hand. Supporting her arm in this way, I'm going to lift her arm. Just after I started to do that, I felt Anne's arm pull slightly inward, away from me. Her muscles retracted and her arm became heavier. I also felt a lessening in the contact between my hand and hers, as if her thought of her arm is of a limb that is shorter than it is. As she reacted in this way, her breathing changed and her torso pulled downward. She tightened in her legs. Since all of this happened, I know that she wasn't inhibiting.

"Anne, let's begin again. This time I'll remind you to inhibit. Take a moment to rise up to your attic. Think of quieting. Think of not lifting your arm. Sustain this thinking as I move you. That's great.

This time I feel that her arm is lighter. It's articulating better in the elbow and shoulder joints. She is allowing me to move her, as her inhibition prevents unnecessary reaction. She's experiencing her arm moving but she isn't overly focused on feelings. Her head, neck, and torso are maintaining a better upward coordination. Her arm is still connected to her back as it moves. Can you perceive these changes, Anne?"

"Yes, you've described a lot of it."

"Great. Now I'm going to put my hand on your midback and another on your hip, but I'm not going to do anything to move you. I'm just going to leave my hands on you as I ask you to sit down in the chair. That's good. Now come back up to standing.

"What did I feel happen as she did this?" I ask as I look out at my audience. "A split second after I asked her to sit, I felt her tighten and pull down in the muscles in her back and abdomen. Her pelvis tilted forward. She also moved back, toward the chair, which meant she pulled herself off balance. The muscles in her legs tightened, making it more difficult for her to bend her legs. Her neck muscles tightened, pulling her head back. In sum, she interfered with her balance and coordination. What can I infer from this about what she was thinking? Her mind seemed to jump ahead of itself to focus on her goal—sitting in the chair. She wasn't inhibiting or directing. Since I'm describing this in words, I have to describe it sequentially. But these aren't a series of separate, isolated events arising from specific and separate parts of her. They're aspects of a whole behavior—her psychophysical habit—the way that she moves, feels, and thinks as she performs the act of sitting. This is a total pattern of activity, which is disconnecting her from herself.

"What set this pattern into action? It was her thought to sit. In a sense my hands enable me to feel backward in time. As I feel her physical response, I can infer something about the mental conception that triggered the action. Her thought began the movement. It is her mental conception of the act of sitting, formed years ago in childhood, that coordinated her body to sit in this particular way. It is this learned mental construct that is the stimulus that produces the action. With my hands on her, I can feel something of this mental concept through what happens in her body as she moves. How can she change how she moves? Through changing this mental conception. Through inhibiting.

"Anne, I'd like you to tell yourself that you're not going to sit. Sustain this thought as I move you slightly back from your ankles. Keep thinking you're not sitting. This doesn't mean that you're preventing me from sitting you. It means that you're inhibiting— you're in your attic, thinking of not sitting, not doing the movement yourself.

"This time I'm feeling that she hasn't jumped ahead, tensing her muscles in an effort to sit. She's allowing me to move her without triggering her reaction. So I know she's inhibiting. I'm also supporting her weight slightly with my hand on her back. My support is allowing her to release the flexor muscles of her torso and legs. This is allowing her torso to lengthen upward. Her pelvis isn't tipping forward. My hands aren't *doing* something to fix her; they're supporting her as she thinks of *not doing*, and so she moves differently. Now I'll bend my legs to lower my body as I continue to support her, and she moves with me. Voilà! Anne is sitting in the chair.

"Did you see the difference in how she did this? Her torso remained more upright. Her leg muscles lengthened, allowing the joints to bend more readily. Her knees bent easily forward; her heels remained on the floor. This didn't happen because I used my hands to make it happen, but because she was inhibiting her interfering habits as I supported and moved her. As a result, now she has experienced the act of sitting in a new, more connected way.

"Next, I'll put my hands on the top of her head and the middle of her back. Anne, think up to your attic as you tell yourself you're not standing. Then think your directions: head forward and up, torso lengthening up and widening, knees forward. Meanwhile, I'm inhibiting and directing myself as I wait to feel how she is changing. Depending on what I perceive, then I make decisions about what to do next with my hands, or what I might say to explain this better.

"Anne, your inhibiting is doing well. Keep thinking of directing your head forward and up. I just felt her head move slightly back. You probably couldn't see it, but I felt it. What does that mean? It means that my student was trying to make her head move forward and up, rather than thinking in the direction forward and up. So I know that her directional thought isn't clear.

"As I've been talking, Anne's neck muscles have released and I feel her forward and up direction. She isn't a beginner. She knows how to inhibit and direct. My hands and words are helping her fine-tune this.

How did I know that she just had a better thought of forward and up? First, she didn't tighten anywhere to make this happen. She didn't pull down in the front of her neck, or under her jaw. Then I felt her head slightly increase its pressure, forward and up, into my hand. Did you perceive that, Anne? What I mean is, could you perceive that you were thinking a more precise forward and up direction?"

"Yes. It's subtle but distinct."

"Good. The information I get from my hands, coupled with my verbal feedback, is teaching her to recognize this change in her thinking and to distinguish these differences. In this way the mental skill of directing becomes much less mysterious.

"Now, think of not standing; direct your head forward and up toward my hand. That's it. I'll move Anne back in the chair while I ask her to continue directing. Let me support your torso with my hand on your back. Sustain the thought of directing your head forward and up toward my hand, then think of lengthening up and widening your back. Think your knees forward, and your heels toward the floor. As I'm talking I'm feeling that this is going well, and I'm directing as well. So I'm going to leave my hands where they are on Anne, and just stand myself up.

"Did you see what happened? Anne sustained her inhibiting and directing while letting me support her, and as I stood up, she rose with me. She didn't react; she didn't try to do it; she didn't hold to her belief of the right way to stand. When the student can think like this, I'm like a waiter carrying a tray in my hand—as I stand she floats up with me, without effort.

"That was great, Anne. You sustained your inhibiting and directing while letting me move you.

"I'll put my left hand on top of Anne's head, and my right hand on the back of her neck and head. Anne, think forward and up. That's good. Now think your torso lengthening up and widening. Think wide in both directions, right and left. That's it. Next, add knees forward—think the direction forward, out in front of you."

"This time I feel she hasn't quite got the forward direction, so I'm going to remember to think my own forward direction. If I'm thinking forward myself, the contact of my hands will help to indicate that to her. That's all I can do. I can't make her think forward."

"I don't know why," Anne interjects, "but forward is a difficult spatial direction for me."

"That's okay. Let it have time. We can wait. Go up to your attic, think of not doing anything. Continue seeing in front of you and building the directions from the beginning, one after the other. I'm waiting, as I also remind myself to think forward.

"That's it, that's a more forward thought. Can you perceive it?" Anne smiles.

"Do you see anything different about her?" I ask the group.

"Her face just changed."

"She looks more present, more alert."

"It looks as though she's here in the room with us and seeing, instead of focusing back inside herself."

"Exactly. She's thinking her directions well. You can see it, particularly in the face and around the eyes."

"Do you notice a change, Anne?"

"When I'm directing forward like this it feels as though I'm standing perilously forward on the edge of a precipice. It's interesting, but it's emotionally uncomfortable. I feel vulnerable. It's different than my usual way of being."

"Yes. Like a lot of us, you lose the forward direction and retreat back inside of yourself. I call it 'being in the back of your cave.'"

Anne smiles, ruefully this time. "That describes it."

"How did you know that her thinking shifted and she had a clearer thought of the forward direction?" someone asks. "She didn't move at all."

"I would say that I was able to feel her thinking change because I was maintaining my own directing. I can't explain how this happens physiologically; I can only describe what it's like as it happens. It seems as if I can sense the change in her inhibiting and directing through my own expanding state of awareness. I knew she was 'back in her cave,' for example, because I experienced some sense of that in myself. Due to my expanding awareness, I seem to experience my inhibiting and directing as well as hers, simultaneously. It sounds odd, but I'm not speaking theoretically. I experience a change in my own state of mind in the present moment. It's just difficult to describe. At this level, knowing what I'm feeling no longer seems to be something that I get from my hands. I seem to sense it in my mind.

"Next, I'm going to put my hands where they were on Anne's torso, ask her to keep directing, and move her some more. I'm gathering information about the specific places where I have my hands, but because I'm maintaining my expanding awareness, I'm also getting a sense of the whole of her—a sense of overall connection, head to neck to torso to limbs as I'm moving her this little bit on her ankles. As I'm moving her there's something bringing my attention to her legs. They don't feel as light and supple as her torso. Where do I *feel* this knowing? It's sort of in my hands, but I think it would be more accurate to say that it's in my overall awareness. I ask myself, What does this tell me about how she's thinking? Is she inhibiting? Is she directing? Is there a particular direction that she's forgetting?

"Anne, I'd like you to think of not tightening, not holding in your legs. Don't go down to your legs to focus on them and feel them. Stay up in your attic and think the words. Let your words have meaning, and let this meaning affect the whole of yourself.

"I've given her some instructions, and I'm waiting to see what I can perceive changing as a result. I feel that her legs have freed a bit. I also feel there's more lightness as I move her. There's a better upward coordination in her torso. Yet something still doesn't feel quite right. It seems to me her legs are doing well, but something keeps telling me there's a problem with her feet. They don't feel as free as her legs. There's something that's just not right about her feet. She's thinking about them differently than she's thinking about the rest of herself."

"That's incredible!" Anne interrupts.

"What?"

"My feet have been hurting a lot lately. I don't know if this is related, but I've been working with a student with a lot of foot problems and I've been thinking about feet. They've really been on my mind recently and they're really bothering me."

I see surprised and wondering faces arrayed before me. "How did I know this?" I ask. "How did I know her feet have been hurting her? I didn't know her feet have been hurting her. Not in the way I know it now, since she just told me. However, in another way I did know it, because my hands and awareness gave me a sense that something about her feet was different from the rest of her. It seemed as though they'd been omitted from her conception of herself.

"I can't explain logically how I knew there was a problem with her feet. It seems impossible, because it's so different from the way we're accustomed to knowing. Let me add that I didn't feel this right away. It took this entire time that I've been working and using my hands. Slowly, I'm increasing what I am able to perceive about the whole of her. Then I had an idea about something interfering with her feet. You tell me how I'm able to know that; I really can't explain it!"

We all have a laugh and I sit Anne down in the chair, since by now she's been standing for a while.

"Let me summarize. You've got to keep your mind quiet and clear, and establish an expanding field of awareness. Do not get distracted by trying to feel the student or yourself. Move your hands to different places and move her. Ask yourself questions; notice contrasts. Ask yourself what you want to know: from specifics, to the overall pattern of movement and beliefs that underlie it, to the student's inhibition and direction. Give your student instructions, notice the changes, and compare them with what you're experiencing in yourself as you inhibit and direct. Gradually, you build an experiential knowledge base—a logbook of sensory understanding. I can't give this knowledge to you, like handing you a manual. There's only one way to acquire it—through sustaining your good psychophysical use of yourself as you teach. Eventually you acquire more and more experience, sensitivity, and understanding.

"However, it's also important to keep in mind that you can be wrong. Do you know for certain that this sense you're having about your student is correct? You can't know you're right in the way you know that it's seventy-two degrees outside when you look at a thermometer. Bells won't go off. There's no one in the teaching room telling you you're right. But when something, whatever it is, keeps nagging at you about what you're sensing, pay attention. Listen and take it in. Then think of ways to test it.

"I sensed something about Anne's feet so I mentioned it. If this had been a lesson, I might have asked her to think of not tightening, or given her some information about how her feet support her weight and contact the floor, and asked her to inhibit by thinking of not standing. Then I'd see if I could feel a change. I wouldn't have told her, directly, 'There's a problem with your feet,' as I did just now. But sometimes when you raise the matter, even indirectly, your student says something that gives you confirmation you're right on target. Then you discover that your hands and awareness can receive information your conscious mind didn't arrive at logically and can't explain.

"Since this knowing seems to come from thin air, we think it's a figment of our imagination. But it's more like a spark jumping the gap—an intuition. It isn't magic. It doesn't come from nowhere. It comes from your years of practice, and your skilled psychophysical use of yourself as you put your hands on the student. Your hands bring you information that is different from your other senses. They bring you another type of knowing. With sufficient practice, your mind learns to understand its meaning."

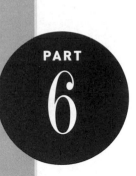

PART

6

CONSCIOUSNESS

OUR NEWEST SENSE

22

Pain Free and Moving Again

An education isn't how much you have committed to memory, or even how much you know. It's being able to differentiate between what you do know and what you don't.

—ANATOLE FRANCE

JOHN, PART TWO

JOHN IS LYING on his back on the table in my teaching room. His knees are bent and his hands rest on his ribs. Several books are positioned under his head to give it support and allow his neck to lengthen. Through his lessons, he is learning to rise up to his attic and to think of non-doing. At the moment, my hands are also helping him to release his hold on his muscles. Slowly his shoulders widen, relinquishing their grip on his chest. The tension in his arms and hands lessens. His palms spread open. Since his inhibiting is improving, I have begun teaching him to think spatially: up, wide, and forward. Today I plan to work more specifically on his original complaint—his painful and stiff right shoulder.

With my left hand under his right elbow, and my other holding his right hand, I extend John's arm at the elbow and support his arm. As I do this, I watch his face for signs of discomfort. I am feeling the response in his muscles and the weight of his arm. My hands bring me a wealth of information as I ask myself questions: Is his arm heavy or light? Are the shoulder, elbow, and wrist mobile or stiff? At the same time, I watch his face: Do his eyes shift downward, losing their brightness as he forgets to aim his attention forward and up? Is he aware of what is around him as he thinks of non-doing? Does he hold his breath? Does he brace in other parts of his body as I move his arm, or does he sustain an overall quality of expansion? These questions and more play across my awareness like tickertape.

Meanwhile, I am paying attention to my own coordination: I let my neck ease to allow my head to move forward and up from my spine. I am thinking my directions. I remind myself not to try to move his arm in a particular way to achieve a result. I wait to feel his muscles' subtle message of release.

"John, does your shoulder hurt as I support your arm away from your side like this?" I ask, checking in.

"No, it's fine."

"Great. Now remember to inhibit and direct. As you bring your attention up to your attic, think of not holding your arm. Think, *I am not lifting my arm*. Then think of letting your head release forward and up from your spine, letting your torso lengthen up and widen, letting your knees release forward from your hips and ankles."

"You know," John interjects, "I wasn't able to let you move my arm like this just a few weeks ago."

"That's right, John. You're doing really well. Think how much you've learned and how much you've changed. And I haven't asked you to do a single exercise!"

John laughs, and then adds, "I'm still worried about my shoulder. It isn't entirely better. Do you think I'll ever be able to get my arm over my head?"

"Yes, but we have to approach this slowly. It isn't good to focus your attention on this single goal. When you do that you stop inhibiting and directing, retriggering the habitual reactions that have created your problem. The important thing isn't how far you move your arm today, it is sustaining your inhibiting and directing as I move you. That's the first step. In the long run that's more valuable. When you become skilled at inhibiting and directing, you can apply these skills in any sit-uation, any time. You'll have gained more than shoulder mobility. Although I don't mean to say that isn't important.

"Remind yourself to rise up to your attic as you think of not moving your arm," I repeat. As I feel the response in John's musculature I move his arm slightly higher. As I do this, I notice John's eyes dropping downward. I feel his arm pulling inward like a turtle retracting a limb into its shell.

"John, where did your attention just go?"

"I guess I'm focused on my arm. I'm feeling what you're doing."

"Good observation. Are you inhibiting as you do that?"

"No," he says, pressing his lips together.

"This is good. You're learning. You noticed that your attention shifted downward to feel. Now renew your inhibition. Think of bringing your attention forward and up, and tell yourself that you're not moving your arm. Then add the directions: my neck is releasing; my head is forward and up; my back is lengthening upward and widening; my knees are forward."

As I speak, I feel John's muscles letting go and I begin to move his arm again. Just as I do this, his eyes drop down and focus inward. His face looks strained; his arm is heavier.

"What are you thinking?" I ask.

"I guess my attention went back to my arm."

"Right. So renew your inhibiting and directing." I wait and watch as John's gaze changes, his facial muscles ease, and his arm becomes responsive in my hands again. Since he is doing well, I begin to rotate his arm, turning it slightly outward in the joint. I wait to feel his muscles release before increasing the range of motion. A moment later something stiffens and tightens. I stop what I'm doing and ask, "What just happened?"

"I'm worrying about what you're doing. I'm worried it's going to hurt."

"Did anything hurt then?"

"No, it really didn't."

I bend John's elbow and bring his arm back to his side, letting his hand rest on his ribs. Then I step back to look at him.

"I'm not very good at this, am I?" he asks, before I have a chance to speak.

"That's not true at all. I just think you have a misapprehension. You're suffering from a pain in your shoulder and lack of mobility in the joint. So you've concluded that your problem is in your shoulder."

"What do you mean?" he asks, slightly startled.

"Well, you're not a refrigerator."

Surprised by my remark, John laughs and answers with feigned innocence, "I'm not?"

"No. But most of us treat ourselves as though we are. Without realizing it, we apply the laws of the external, inanimate world to our body. When the refrigerator breaks, what do you do? You have to figure out what's broken, and then you have to get a new part, replacing the old one. In other words, you have to figure out what's wrong, and then know the right thing to do to fix it. But you don't work that way. You're not a bunch of parts. You're a living organism, a complex array of interdependent and interacting systems. You can't just take your arm off and put on a new one."

"No," he says, smiling again.

"For example, your body knows how to heal itself. When you cut your finger it heals, right? You don't know, consciously, how to do that. Yet you treat your arm as though it's your job to focus on it as if it were a broken part for you to fix. You have a belief that if you really focus on that arm you'll be able to feel what's wrong, and then do the right thing to make it get better. But that's not possible. In addition, while you focus so much on the pain in your shoulder, you neglect to notice what is happening in the rest of your body and around you. Am I right?"

"Yeah, I am pretty focused on this."

"Because of this belief—that by focusing on feeling your arm you'll know what to do—you're reacting to your pain in a way that makes the pain worse. The stimulus of pain is gradually teaching your brain to overfocus its attention on feeling the part of your body from which the pain seems to arise. It is also triggering your brain to believe that you're in danger. Your brain responds to this pain as a threat, stimulating a defense response that leads to all sorts of changes in your neurochemistry. You begin producing stress hormones. Other physical changes are triggered throughout your body as well that create more tension in your muscles. This is a stress response. In turn, it creates more pain.

"Your locomotor system and your self-defense system are interlinked. Over time, in a sense you acquire two injuries: the painful, stiff shoulder, and the way that you have learned to overfocus your attention on feeling the shoulder. You are unwittingly retriggering and compounding this defense response. In order to recover, we have to deal with both: the injury and the way you've learned to react to it. What do you think the remedy for this is? Exercising your muscles more?"

"No," John says. "Inhibiting?"

"You've got it. Want to try this again?"

"Sure."

I hold John's arm at the elbow and hand, and extend his arm outward from his side. Then I stop, ask him to rise up to his attic and think of not doing anything with his arm, and then to think up, wide, and forward. "Remind yourself not to focus on feeling your arm. I know it's scary, since you're afraid of having pain, but ask yourself to think and behave as if the arm isn't injured. In this way you can indirectly prevent your fear reaction. You can think as if you believe your arm is okay. This allows you a new way of responding as I move you."

Watching John's expression, I see that he understands what I'm saying. "That's good, John. Keep thinking forward and up to your attic. Then try thinking, 'I don't have to fix my arm.'"

John's arm begins to lengthen and lighten in my hands. I slowly rotate the arm outwardly, but in the next instant his attention pulls inward again. I stop what I'm doing and continue to support his arm. "John, think of rising up to your attic. From your attic your awareness can expand to think of the whole of yourself, not just your shoulder and arm. Remember, you're not a bunch of parts. We want your thinking to encompass the whole of you. From up in your attic you can be aware of the whole—head to fingers to toes. You're thinking of *not* dwelling on your fears and feelings, as you allow me to move you just a bit."

As I'm speaking, John's arm is beginning to lengthen again. I'm able to rotate it outwardly a little more. As this happens, muscles release around his scapula and in his back. This enables me to move his arm higher over his head. John's hand is about six or seven inches above his shoulder. I know this is farther than it has moved in quite a while. I stop moving it but continue supporting his arm as I wait. John is inhibiting and directing, and seeing out in front of him without focusing on his arm. He is sustaining a more balanced attention and awareness of the whole of himself.

"John, that's good. You're thinking more of the whole, can you tell? Do you sense what I mean by that? You're no longer just 'an injured arm' in your awareness, am I right?"

"Yes, I can sense the difference. I'm less focused on my arm and what you're doing."

"Great. You're changing your habit of mind–body disconnection. Continue aiming your attention forward and up to your attic. This allows an awareness of the whole of yourself to emerge, instead of focusing on just a part. I'm supporting and moving your arm, but your job is to think of not doing anything, and then think up, wide, and forward. That's great." John's muscles lengthen as I slowly move his arm higher. Then I stop, wait a moment, then move his arm even more upward. His shoulder muscles continue to release, his back muscles lengthen, and his arm is light and mobile.

"John, continue that good thinking. Now in addition, can you let yourself be peripherally aware of where your arm is?"

"It's higher?"

"I'll say it is. Your hand is about two feet higher than your shoulder joint. It's almost straight over your head. Does anything hurt?"

"No, not at all. This is incredible. My arm hasn't moved like this in over a year. How did you do that? How did this happen?" Questions tumble out as a wondering smile spreads across his face.

"I'm not doing this, John, you are. I can't move your arm in a way that you don't allow me to. I can't make your muscles let go. It's your thought that is doing this. You're inhibiting, so your muscles are letting go. But you're not just releasing some muscles; you're letting go of beliefs, preventing fear reactions, and changing old habits of over-focusing your attention on sensation. You're also thinking spatially, which is restoring a headward coordination in the muscles of your torso. Your thinking is allowing the whole of you to lengthen and expand, not just your arm. Can you tell?"

"This is amazing," he repeats. "And I'm not doing anything," he adds in a voice that sounds more like a question than a statement.

"Well, you're not doing anything in the sense that you're no longer holding on to your muscles. But you're learning to sustain your thinking in a new and beneficial way. This is what you're here to learn, not just how to fix your arm. You're not a refrigerator, remember? You're a thinking, responding, learning, interactive whole. The way you move affects how you think. How you think affects how you move, which affects how you feel. If you change one, you'll change them all. Instead of reacting to your arm in a way that hinders and limits you, mentally and physically, you're learning to think in a way that frees you from learned belief, tension, and fear. That's what we want, isn't it?

"Most people's unconscious habits take them in a direction of ever-increasing tension, fear, and rigidity as they age. But it doesn't have to be that way. You don't have to stiffen and become less mobile. You don't have to become fixed in your behaviors and beliefs. You can learn to inhibit and direct, to use these tools to enable you to change and respond ever more appropriately and adaptively in each moment, and to play a greater role in maintaining and optimizing your health."

John is silent for a moment as I bend his arm and place his hand back in its resting position on his ribs. Then he turns his head toward me. "I'm getting a lot more from these lessons than I expected."

I smile and nod.

"I really didn't expect this was going to work," he continues. "A friend of mine nagged me to try it, so I called you to get him off my back. I figured I'd be able to tell him that I tried it and it was a lot of nonsense. I didn't believe this would work!"

23

An Incredible Lightness of Being

The purpose of education is to replace
an empty mind with an open one.
—MALCOLM FORBES

ERIN, PART THREE

Erin has had five months of weekly lessons. She is learning what it means to inhibit as she sits and stands, allowing me
to move her. She is also learning to direct, and has become familiar with my vocabulary and what is required of her as a partic-
ipant in the lesson. At the moment, she is sitting on the chair in
my teaching room, and I am standing on her left side. My right
hand is placed on the back of her neck and head.

"Erin, think of directing—let your head release forward and
up, your torso lengthen upward and widen, and your knees
release forward." As I speak, I feel a sinking quality at the base
of Erin's neck. With a glance in the mirror, I see that she is looking downward. She has responded to my instructions by dropping her attention down to feel her body. From this, I know she
is doing something in her body in an effort to think.

"Let's make this simpler, Erin. Think up to your attic and see
out in front of you. Take time to quiet the chatter in your
mind." I pause, taking time for her to absorb my words. "Think

of not sitting. Think of not doing anything to help me. Say these words silently to yourself as you summon their meaning in your mind. You want to know what you mean by these words." As I wait, I feel a quality of calm spread through Erin like leaves settling as the wind stills. The downward pressure in her neck has lifted.

"That's good, Erin. Can you tell that you're thinking more clearly?"

"Yes."

"Now add your spatial thinking. First think up, toward and beyond your head." I put my left hand lightly on top of Erin's head. "Think in the direction that is toward my hand that's on top of your head. Let your words summon the meaning of expansion upward, to the top of your head and beyond. This is just a thought, an effortless thought. You're not trying to do anything to your body." I pause while my hands bring me information about how Erin has responded to my instruction. She feels more focused and clear, easier in her body yet not relaxed. She also feels more energized, and I can move her more readily.

"Now add the widening thought—think of expanding out your ears. Wide is the direction of elevator doors sliding open." Again, I wait.

"Add a thought of forward—expanding into the space in front of you."

As I speak, I feel Erin's response. She understands my instructions. My hands feel her head releasing slightly forward and up, away from her neck. Her neck seems to soften and fill. Her shoulders release apart and away from her ribs. Her torso is coordinating headward. As I move her slightly forward and backward from her hips, she feels light yet strong—mobile, yet connected through her pelvis into the chair.

"That's good. You're inhibiting and directing rather than focusing on feeling things in yourself and trying to do the right thing to your body. Can you notice a difference in your thinking?"

Erin nods her head. Since this is going well, I put her directing skill to a greater test. Applying a small pressure into the heel of my palm as it rests on the base of her neck, I extend my arm to pivot Erin farther forward in the chair. I have made no mention of standing up, but in an instant Erin changes. Her legs tighten and pull inward. There is a downward compression in her torso. She no longer feels buoyant. In reaction to the sensation of moving, Erin's brain has jumped into action, tensing muscles in her legs, abdomen, and lower back. I move her to the upright.

"What happened to your thinking?" I ask.

"I don't know, it just sort of disappeared."

"Tell yourself not to react to the feeling of the movement. Just think of not standing. Remember, I'll do the job of moving you. Your job is to inhibit and renew your directions—let your head release forward and up, your torso lengthen up and widen, your knees release forward. Think these directions to yourself, one after the other and all together. You don't have to think about doing the movement itself."

Erin doesn't reply, but I know through my hands that she is resuming her spatial thinking. She is lengthening upward. Her torso feels more supple and toned. I move her forward again. This time as she moves Erin continues directing. Instead of her torso sinking away from my hand as she pivots forward, she seems to rise up into my hand. Her muscles lengthen; her spine extends upward. Her legs do not grip or pull her knees together. Next I move her backward toward the upright, but in an instant the sinking in her body returns. What a moment before had felt lively, vibrant, and springy under my hand now seems to have withdrawn and sunk inward.

"Did you notice any change in your spatial thinking just then?"

"Yes," she answers, "As you moved me backward I thought about my bottom on the chair."

"Were you thinking spatially?" I ask.

"No!" She replies with energy.

"Which direction would you say you lost?"

"Forward. I started thinking back, toward the chair."

"Okay, great. Let's try it again." I repeat the directions to her and with guidance from my hand she moves forward again.

"Continue directing, Erin. Allow your thought of up, wide, and forward to expand into the space around you." I move her torso to the upright once again.

"That's the idea. Could you perceive a difference this time?"

"I just kept thinking my directions. It seemed lighter."

"Right. That's a good clue that your directing is working. It coordinates you in a way that lets your body lighten; it loses its quality of weight. Just don't get caught up in focusing on the feeling. You can be peripherally aware of it, but the important thing is to sustain your inhibiting and directing."

Next, I move my right hand to her midback. My left hand is still on top of her head. I resume thinking my own directions and, as I lengthen through my arms, I begin to add the slightest increasing pressure from my left hand into her head. By doing this I am testing the waters again. If she is inhibiting and directing, this slight increase of pressure will cause her to respond with an increasing tonus in the muscles of her back, which will make her torso rise upward. Otherwise, my pressure on her head will send her downward. She will shorten and move away from my contact. I remind Erin to think forward and up. I feel her head dropping down. Her chin tucks into her neck and her neck flattens.

"Think in the direction that is toward my hand on your forehead, Erin. Think your head forward and up." I feel her head starting to pull slightly backward. "That's not up, Erin. Which way is up? You're thinking back and up, not forward and up. Think forward and up toward my hand." After a moment she shifts again. Her head rights itself on the top of her neck and her torso lengthens. Her chin releases away from her neck and her neck regains its soft, expanding quality.

"That's good. Now your directing is better. Can you tell?"

"Yes, but it is such a slight change!"

I increase the pressure slightly on Erin's head again, as I also increase the pressure of my right hand on her back. With this slight increase in contact against her back and head simultaneously as she directs, there is a subtle but marvelous shift. As my hands move slightly inward toward each other, Erin expands outward, toward my hands. Her back widens and frees upward. Her ribs move more readily. Her head frees forward on her spine, as it seems to reach into my palm. It feels as though I'm holding a coiled spring that is expanding outward against my palms.

Since this is going well, I move my arms to the right, this time moving Erin so she is pivoting back in the chair from her hip joints. In the next instant her body has become heavier again. I respond by increasing the contact of my right hand on her back to give her more support. In order to do this, I continue directing so that I meet her weight with my own length and expansion, especially through my back and legs. This gives me more strength so that I can support her without tightening and pulling downward in myself.

As I sustain this greater contact, I feel that Erin's abdominal muscles have lengthened and her ribs are moving. She is breathing

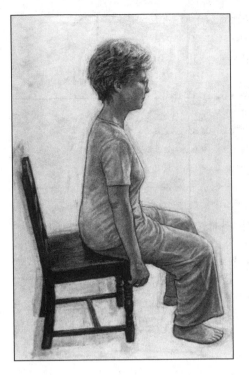

23-1. Erin sitting. Her neck tension has eased. Her head is forward and up, and her back muscles have released to allow her spine to coordinate upward. The shoulders are wide apart and the arms hang freely. Her knees are not squeezed together; her leg muscles have lengthened.

better. As this happens her body frees upward again, releasing into lightness and buoyancy. The spring returns beneath my hands. Sustaining this now for about thirty seconds, I know she has accomplished a lot. I move Erin to the vertical and take my hands off her (Illustration 23-1).

"That was great, Erin. "You kept inhibiting and directing as I moved you back in the chair. My hand on your back was also giving you support as I moved you. This allowed your abdominal muscles to release, which freed your torso to lengthen more upward. We work together as a team: your inhibition and direction, my support and gentle hands-on guidance as I move you. If you hadn't been inhibiting and directing, we both would have had to work a lot harder as you moved back in space.

"Ready to try this again?" Erin nods. "Remember that you don't have to move your body. Moving your body is my job. You're rising up to your attic, and then inhibiting and directing. Don't zero in on the sensation of the movement. It's directing you want to give your attention to, not the physical body that you believe you have to hold on to and figure out how to move. Think spatially in all dimensions: up, wide, and forward." I place my hands again on her head and back. "And think forward and up, releasing toward my hand on your head as I move you. This time I'll move you a bit farther back in the chair."

I begin to move Erin back, but she begins to shrink downward again.

Before I can say anything she says, "I lost it. My mind wandered."

"That's good. You noticed when you stopped thinking. When that happens, you have the opportunity to restore it. That's how you practice and build your skill." I bring Erin to the upright as I leave my hands on her back and head. We try again.

This time Erin sustains her thinking. It feels as if I have a spring between my hands. As I gently press my hands against this spring, continuing to direct and lengthen in myself, she releases and expands into my hands. Now I do not simply have light hands, delicately touching my student. I have strong, spreading hands that make fuller contact, yet I am not tensing my muscles to try to hold her or do something to her by grasping her with my fingers. I expand as my muscles lengthen, as though I am a rubber band being stretched and gaining in tensile strength. As I meet her weight and she meets my hand, the dynamic expansion between us increases the muscle tone in both of us. Together, we are becoming longer and stronger while also light, free, and mobile.

I move my hand to the back of Erin's head and neck. I continue moving her forward in the chair, then backward, then forward again. By doing this I can feel how she is sustaining her thinking in response to my instruction. I can feel that she is listening and understanding. She is no longer focusing on her body and trying to do the right thing. Her back widens as she moves. Her limbs are strong, yet mobile. She moves with virtually no effort. It is as if her torso is glued to my hand and, since I am moving, she moves also. As we do this, her head reorients on the top of her spine, pivoting slightly forward on the top of her neck. The musculature in her abdomen releases a little more. This allows her lower ribs to continue freeing, expanding more to bring air into her lungs, then moving together on the exhalation. Her body seems to have lost its mass and become open space.

When her torso is about eight or ten inches behind the vertical, I stop moving. I can feel that Erin is directing. She is lengthening outward and into my hands; I am lengthening in my hands, arms, back, and legs. I repeat the directions to her again, asking her to aim her thought in the direction that is forward and up. As she does this I can feel a greater connection through her whole body, from her head to the bottom of her spine and into her legs and feet to the floor. She feels whole. My support also enables Erin to lengthen her hip flexor muscles, and this allows her torso to lengthen further upward, releasing her previously downward compression. I think my directions, particularly forward and up. I increase the contact, reminding myself to allow the increasing force of this contact to travel through my arm, back, legs, and into the floor.

As sure as I will ever be that we are both directing, I straighten my legs and stand myself up, simultaneously moving my arms in a sideward and up direction. Because Erin is also directing, she feels weightless. She moves as if her joints are frictionless. Her torso is vertical as she rises up out of the chair like a rocket in liftoff. At the

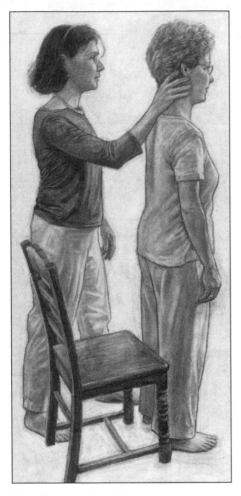

23-2. Erin standing with better balance and more upward coordination in the torso. Contrast this with Illustration 14-1.

moment I have finished and am standing, my student is also standing, poised and balancing upright with ease (Illustration 23-2).

I take my hand off her as Erin's head swivels toward me and an astonished grin spreads across her face. "How'd that happen?" she blurts out. "I didn't do that! You lifted me up out of the chair, right? How'd you do that? I didn't stand up!" her questions tumble out. I smile but say nothing.

My student looks happily perplexed as she repeats, "How did you lift me out of the chair?"

I shake my head. "I didn't. I didn't lift you. You did it. Or rather we should say your thinking did it."

"Are you sure?" she asks again. "That was astonishing. I felt like I was a bird, expanding outward through my limbs until I—"

Erin stops, searching for words.

"I let go of my body and flew!"

24

Speaking from My Self

The voice is a second signature.

—R. I. FITZHENRY

GREG

NOT LONG AGO, a young man named Greg called me for lessons. He had recently completed college as a theater major. Tall and handsome, with dark hair and chiseled features, Greg sat in the chair in my teaching room and assured me he had no pains or injury.

"What is your interest in the Technique?" I asked.

"I keep finding references to it in my acting textbooks. And friends keep telling me how useful it is for actors. I thought I should try it."

"You're right. It is helpful for actors. Among other things, it helps prevent you from being typecast. Most of us have an unconscious way of holding and moving our body. We usually aren't aware of it, but it conveys a certain personality type. As a result, when you audition, you find yourself being given the same types of roles. The Technique can teach you to prevent these habits and learn to move in a more neutral way. Then you can add on to this whatever movements and mannerisms best suit your character. You'll be more able to convey a range of characters and emotions."

Greg smiled and assured me that this was what he wanted.

Over the next several months, Greg arrived punctually for his weekly lessons. He smiled easily, but he also seemed constrained. In his early lessons, I discovered that this ready smile belied a different inner state. Greg's body was extremely tight. It was hard work lifting and moving his arms and legs as he rested on the table. I found myself wondering how he had managed in his movement classes.

I continued working with him on the table more than I had intended. Greg needed to learn to inhibit, and the best way to teach him this was to let him lie on the table, where he did not have to hold himself up against gravity.

Gradually, Greg began to change. His too-ready smile lessened. His limbs became lighter and easier to move. He looked more graceful as he walked. Each week at the end of the lesson, he said that he found the lessons helpful. I believed him but he never said more specifically what he meant by this.

One day as Greg was lying on the table and inhibiting, I commented on how much he had changed since his first lesson.

"I'll say," Greg answered quickly in an odd tone of voice. "I don't feel so much like smashing heads anymore."

Greg's remark took my breath away as I struggled to think of a response. "Great," was all I could think to say.

As I thought over his comment later, I was puzzled. Greg had a friendly, outgoing manner. He smiled, laughed, and chatted during the lessons, although I had soon learned how tense his body was. But "feeling like smashing heads"? This spoke of a different level of tension. And it spoke of distress. I did not believe that he would actually do this, or feel myself in danger, but I began to understand Greg a bit more. He was letting me know something of the enormity of his inner struggle. And I had a new appreciation for the extent of Greg's tension. He must be living, I realized, locked within his body so tightly that this created a feeling, and an accompanying belief, that the only way to break out of this tension was to explode, violently. And all the while, Greg had no idea why he felt this way or what to do about it. He just kept smiling, wearing his mask of joviality. This must have been tiring and alienating. Greg was a young man split within himself.

Although I was startled by his remark, I felt gratified to realize that the lessons were helping to release him from this inner struggle. As Greg's body continued to ease, I began working with him in the chair. One day I decided to begin building a bridge between what he was learning in the lessons and his acting. As he sat in the chair, I asked him if he would like to read something out loud.

Greg's eyes widened as he answered, "Sure!"

I handed him a copy of da Vinci's *Notebooks* and asked him to pick a page and read. Greg opened the book and began. I watched and listened with surprise. As a trained actor, I had expected his voice to command a certain presence. But Greg's voice was muted and flat. There was no resonance. He sounded lifeless. Occasionally he would emphasize one word more than the next, but his voice had a disembodied quality as though there was no living person behind it. I asked him to stop reading and put the book in his lap.

"What were you thinking as you read, Greg, can you say?"

"Not really. Well, I guess I was actually thinking about pronouncing the words correctly."

"What about the meaning of your words? Did you follow what it was you were reading?"

"No, I wasn't paying attention to that."

"Try it again."

Greg read a few paragraphs, but it was the same as before. His voice was stilted. I found myself barely able to follow what he was saying. "Okay, Greg, stop." As he put the book down, I asked, "What were you thinking this time? Did you notice anything else?"

"Well, I was trying to read the words correctly," he repeated.

"What about you? Where was Greg as he was reading?"

"Me?"

"Yes. Were you aware of yourself?"

"No, not at all."

"Where did *you* go?"

Greg dropped his eyes; he seemed to be studying the book in his lap. "I don't know."

"You are important, Greg. You aren't just a voice reading some words on a page, disconnected from the person that is you. You are allowed to get into the act. It is okay to be aware of yourself as you read. And it is okay for you to think about the meaning of the words you're reading and be affected by them. You can allow yourself to get into the scene, so to speak.

"Try this again, but this time, before you begin, let me ask you to take a moment to be aware of yourself as you are sitting on the chair, and of your feet on the floor, and the space around you. Then inhibit and direct. Now see if you can sustain some of this awareness of yourself, and your thinking, as you read. Give it a try." As I speak I am kneeling next to Greg. My hand is on his back, allowing me to feel his response to my instructions.

Greg lifts the book. He pauses a moment and begins to read. This time his voice has more fullness, a little more variation of expression. After a while I ask him to stop and tell me what he has noticed.

Greg is silent, searching for something to say. "Well, I was a bit more aware of myself. I noticed myself holding the book. I was thinking my directing, as you asked." Greg pauses. "Actually, I was kind of worried."

"What about, can you say?"

"I really have my mind on trying to say the words correctly."

"That's a good observation. We'll do this again, but first let me help you a little. Bring the book up in front of you. Hold it higher, in front of your face." I guide Greg's arm upward as my other hand rests lightly on his back. "Take a moment to be aware of seeing the words on the page. Don't strain to see them, or zoom in to focus on them, just be aware of seeing. You can also see what's around the book as well, on either side of the pages. Do you follow me?"

"Yeah."

"As you're seeing, remind yourself that you don't have to leave yourself out of the picture as you focus on the words. You want to be present, in this time and space, sitting on this chair. As you look at the page, be aware that the light is bringing the words to you. The light bounces off the page and passes through the lens in your eyes where it is focused, and then stimulates the cells at the back of your eyes. Those cells transform the light into nerve signals that are sent to the back of your brain. It's a misnomer to say that you're reading the words on the page. You're reading the words as your brain processes these signals in your visual cortex at the back of your head. Reading doesn't happen out there. It happens inside YOU.

"Also, take as much time as you need as you're reading. We're in no rush."

Greg begins to read again. This time a new timbre and resonance has come into his voice. I notice that he is breathing better. His arm seems lighter as he is holding the book. The tension in his shoulders and back has eased.

"Okay, Greg, now stop. That was different, could you tell?"

"Yeah, I felt better. I wasn't trying so hard to read the words. I sort of let them come to me."

"That's great. You seemed calmer. Your voice was fuller." Keeping my hand on his back, I put my other hand on the top of his head. "Leave the book on your lap for now and take a moment to think of rising up to your attic. That's good. From here you can be more aware of the whole of yourself, head to fingers to toes." I pivot Greg's torso slightly forward and back as I speak, and feel an improving connection from his head to his neck and spine.

"That's good, Greg. Now think your directions—you're up in your attic, aware of yourself. You're thinking of your head releasing forward and up from your neck, of your back lengthening up and widening, of your legs releasing forward away from your torso. Add a thought of not tensing your jaw. Try again."

As Greg reads, I use my hands to move his torso slightly back and forth, assisting him to lengthen more upward. I turn his head and neck slightly, encouraging mobility. His reading is going well, but then suddenly something shifts. Greg's body seems to lock. I can't move him. His focus seems to have shrunk inward and there's a break in his voice. He stops reading in the middle of a sentence. "What were you thinking?"

"I got confused about that word. I was worrying about how to say it."

"Did you notice what else happened to you when you were worrying about your pronunciation?"

"I got tense?"

"Right. What else happened?"

"It happened so fast I'm not sure, but I had a thought that I wouldn't be able to pronounce it correctly. Then I felt my neck and jaw get tense. When I felt that, I focused even harder on the page. I completely lost my awareness and thinking. Then I stumbled on the word. I also felt bad. It's upsetting. I got this knot in my stomach. It's still there."

"You're making important observations, Greg. Isn't it amazing how much can go on inside yourself in such a brief moment in time?"

"I'll say."

"Do you want to do this some more?"

"Yeah, this is interesting."

"Take time to restore your thinking. Rise up to your attic. Allow an awareness of yourself to come alive within you. Even that queasy feeling in your stomach, that is part of what is happening in yourself in the moment. You don't have to get rid of it. That feeling isn't the enemy or a problem. Let it be. If you don't battle with it, trying to get rid of it, it'll disappear on its own. And even if you stumble on a word, that's part of what's happening within you in the present moment. It's real. It isn't bad. You haven't failed when this happens. Everybody does it. And since this triggers a reaction in you, a psychophysical reaction, as an actor you can use that to your advantage. That's something you want to allow to happen in yourself. When emotion rises within you it affects your voice. That's good. That's what you want. The listener hears the emotion in your sound and is affected by it.

"You don't have to try to sound a certain way, or put something deliberately into your expression. Just let it happen within you as you experience the meaning of the words you're speaking, and are affected by their meaning. You don't want to cut yourself off from yourself as you feel things happening inside you—as a person or as an actor. Let the meaning and the experience affect you. You don't have to control and manage what happens."

Greg begins again. This time his voice comes more readily. His voice is lighter and more expressive. After a few moments of reading, however, his voice reverts to its old flatness. His voice tells me that Greg has disappeared again. He stops reading.

"How about this time? What happened?"

"I lost it again. Everything I was thinking about evaporated."

"Any idea why?"

"Well," he says slowly, "This feels so different from the way I usually read."

"How?"

"This is making me realize how much I shut myself down. I really turn myself off. I guess it's because reading this way feels pretty overwhelming. I'm feeling so many things. It feels so vulnerable."

"Do you want to stop?"

Greg shakes his head.

"This time, as you read, remind yourself that you are the one who is reading and you are essential to this process. No matter how it feels, just continue renewing your decision to rise up to your attic and become aware of the whole of yourself. Think of inhibiting your reaction to those uncomfortable feelings. These are just sensations. Let them rise up within you and then pass through you. You can say no to your habit of cutting yourself off, shutting yourself out of the picture.

"Be aware of yourself and be affected by what you're reading and by the changes that happen within you as you read. It isn't your job to make your voice sound a certain way. It's your job to read, and to allow the meaning of the words to rise within you and affect you. Let yourself be affected; let yourself be surprised. You can't predetermine how this will turn out." I take my hands off Greg and move away.

Greg nods his head, picks up the book and begins to read. Shortly afterward I feel the hair on my arms stand on end. I feel a lump rising in my throat. Greg's voice is entirely different. Something seems to have risen within him and emerges, unexpected, unedited, unconstrained. His voice has presence, color, and resonance. As he continues, his rhythm changes as well. He pauses more often, yet as the listener I am entranced. The silence communicates something, too. I find myself taking in the meaning of his words as he speaks. Images spring to mind. His voice is more complete, more whole. There is expressiveness in his voice but it doesn't sound contrived. It sounds authentic, born of the meaning of his words as they resonate within him. Greg looks free and easy in his body. His breath comes in and out more readily. His voice is alive.

Greg stops, puts the book down and looks up at me. "Wow."

"Greg, that was terrific. You gave me goose bumps. What was different, can you say? What were you thinking?"

"I thought about the meaning of the words. And I thought of myself, and let the words affect me. I stopped reacting to my worry. I let it be. I had to stop once in a while to get clear about the meaning; sometimes I lost it. When I read so that I could understand the words, I didn't worry about what you were thinking or whether I was saying them correctly. I felt more connected with myself." He pauses. "I didn't know it could be like that."

"I don't know if you perceived it, Greg, but I can give you the feedback that your voice was entirely different. It had expressiveness, but it didn't sound as though you were trying to make it be expressive. It flowed out of you. I also understood what you were saying better. The pauses weren't a problem because I was right there with you. When you stopped to understand the meaning, it gave me time to understand it as well. It was wonderful. You read just a few paragraphs but I was so moved. "

Greg's eyes drop and he shakes his head as he says, "Why didn't they teach me this in acting class?" Then he looks up at me, his eyes bright. "That was so great. I feel like such a different person. I feel more connected to myself. I feel more whole. Do you know what I mean?"

25

Self-Mastery:
Connnection

The whole problem is to establish
communication with one's self.
——E. B. WHITE

I F WE LOOK around us and take a moment to notice our
behavior and beliefs, we see that a split pervades our thinking
and our lives. We are plagued by division: east-west, nature-nur-
ture, liberal-conservative, science-religion, true-false, subjective-
objective, good-bad, heaven-hell, body-mind. Are these an
inevitable part of the fabric of nature and life itself, or are they perhaps an outer projection of an inner flaw, a hairline fracture in the
lens through which we conceptualize ourselves and our world?

This split thinking pervades our medical system, school system, political system, social fabric, and cultural identity. Usually,
our efforts to solve the problems this way of thinking creates only
cause further separation: First we take apart and then we take our
stand, defending one side while we attack, denigrate, or deny the
other. We spend our lives standing on one side or the other of
so many dividing lines that we fail to recognize this as a symptom of a deeper problem. The truth of our self-dividing lens
never comes into our awareness.

What is this split vision? Why is it so difficult to recognize?
Can it be joined? Can we learn to conceive of ourselves, and to

behave not only with better balance and coordination, but also with greater *connection*?

I have likened our sixth sense, bodily sensation, to a mirror in the mind that gives us a view into the realm of our psychophysical being. It is from this sense, more than any of our others, that our mind generates an organizing matrix, a conception of a "self" that "behaves." I also suggested that it is our capacity for language that acts as a second mirror facing the first, allowing us to reflect on this self: to create an increasingly complex construct that forms opinions and beliefs, thinks about what is happening to itself, makes judgments and choices, and describes its experiences through the added reflection of symbolic language.

Our brain's ability not only to interpret and misinterpret sensory data but to synthesize this data into a self-picture on which we can reflect could be called our capacity for *self-consciousness*—which, although scientists cannot agree on its definition or explain exactly how we do it, no one disputes that we possess. Further, this very consciousness of self acts as yet another sensory system, a *supra* sensory system (an eighth sense) capable of generating stimuli that drive our behavior and affect the functioning of the whole organism. *Thus, consciousness-of-self is both a construct of the individual and an active player upon the individual.*

Self-consciousness is often thought of as something fixed, an attribute that exists within us like our ability to digest food. It is equated simply with being awake. But it is much more than this. Let us imagine our consciousness-of-self as a sort of hologram in the mind, shifting and changing with every new input to or change in the organism. It is a *potentiality* within us, not an object or a trait. Through it we can learn to become ever more self-aware. This self-consciousness holds the key to unlocking many of our inner mysteries, enabling us to learn new skills and to change our psychophysical behavior in healthful and beneficial ways. *This hologram of the self can enhance the organism from which it arises.*

As we have seen, however, there are many factors that can damage, distort, and splinter this gossamer construction of self-consciousness. Danger—real or perceived—is a primary source of trouble as the organism acts to mount its defense but in so doing often seems to tear itself apart in pain and fear. Another critical element is our unconscious misuse of our locomotor system, which generates bodily feedback that warps the primary mirror through which we see ourselves.

Herein lies our dilemma: If the lens of self-vision has become distorted, how can we see its flaw? How can we know that it needs correction?

In a serendipitous moment, Alexander simply used another mirror. Through it, he observed himself (from outside looking in) and saw his divide. He saw that he was not doing what he thought he was doing; that he was not able to stop doing what he did not want to do; that his *way of thinking* determined how he acted; and that his *way of moving* led to faulty self-judgments and beliefs. It seemed that his self-consciousness, the hologram in his mind, was operating the dials of the machine that had created it, but in so doing was damaging the machine itself. In turn, the machine was further distorting the hologram. Creation and creator had been split apart, and each was harming the other. He was caught in a wheel of distortion, self-delusion, and further distortion.

But looking in the mirror, Alexander also saw the fundamental unity of himself. All of his parts acted on all the others. He was not a collection of pieces that could be treated separately. He was a psychophysical whole, and only a psychophysical approach could get to the root of his problem. Both the machine and the hologram needed repair simultaneously. Through meticulous self-experimentation, Alexander learned to change his way of thinking by inhibiting his psychophysical reactions. And he learned to change his way of moving by directing to restore his balance and coordination. These changes generated new sensory feedback as he moved and as he acted, which restored a truer self-perception. Gradually the disparate and damaged parts of himself were reconnected and repaired. Hologram and machine were no longer divided and in conflict but reconnected. Alexander had created an applied methodology that healed the breach within.

These observations and experiences led him to theorize that humans are evolving in a direction of increasing self-consciousness. He viewed this as a potential within each of us waiting to be developed. He saw that this potential existed along a continuum. It was possible to be more or less conscious, to be more or less a victim of our self-distortion. It remained for each of us to choose to act to become *skillfully* self-conscious.

Alexander believed this potential must be developed for the betterment of the individual, and also for humankind. He thought civilization was in serious peril due to our one-sided focus on acquiring knowledge about everything except ourselves, and for too often being wrong when convinced we are right.

Alexander did not care for grand theories of consciousness and human betterment. What use were theories without a practical method that demonstrably succeeded? He knew he had developed such a method. He had demonstrated that the skills of inhibition and direction could be consciously learned, enabling each person to self-correct, and thus to overcome many of the ills that "our flesh is heir to." He dreamed that one day we would all be able to draw from this knowledge, overcoming the split within, and realizing our gift for conscious self-connection and self-mastery.

G and H

He who chooses the beginning of a road
chooses the place it leads to.
—HARRY EMERSON FOSDICK

G HOW TO STRENGTHEN YOUR BACK

To arrive at the simple is difficult.
—RASHID ELISHA

IN SECTION A, you learned how to rest your back muscles by lying in semisupine and in the prone position. In this section you will lie in prone as you do the opposite activity—strengthening your back muscles—specifically, the deep back muscles of your primary locomotor system.

After years of misuse as we sit, stand, and perform our daily activities, the superficial muscles of the back become excessively tight and the deep muscles of the back become weak. The way that most people exercise reinforces this imbalance. In addition, many people believe that it is the abdominal muscles—not the back muscles—that should be strengthened. They typically do sit-ups, further compounding their malcoordination. It is the deep muscles of the back that should support your head and trunk when you are upright, not your abdominal muscles.

I do not usually recommend strengthening exercises for specific muscles, but this exercise is important because so many of us are weak in this area. As you have probably begun to appreciate however, there is no exercise that can guarantee success, because any exercise can be performed badly. Do not practice this while your mind is wandering. The benefits of this activity depend on how you think as you move. To strengthen the deep muscles of your back effectively, you must inhibit and direct.

Please read the instructions and the following discussion before beginning.

Neck Extensors

[Note: If you have a neck injury, or neck or shoulder pain, do not try this without the assistance of an Alexander teacher.]

1. Lie in prone with a book or pillow under your sternum. (Review this position in Illustration A-2-1.) Place your arms on the floor at your sides, palms up, with your elbows bent. Alternatively, you may rest your arms on the floor with your hands above your head, palms on the floor, elbows bent, and your upper arms away from your body. (See Illustration G-2-1.) Let your upper forehead contact the floor. Let your shoulders fall forward toward the floor. Bring your attention up to your attic. Think, *I am* not *tensing my neck,* or *I am* not *tensing my muscles.*

2. The very small movement you will be doing is lifting your neck so that it moves slightly back—toward the ceiling—away from the floor. As your neck moves back it will also lift your head slightly off the floor (Illustration G-1-1) .

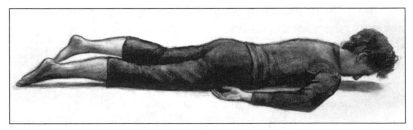

G-1-1. Prone: lifting the neck back using the neck extensors, which raises the head slightly off the floor.

First, rise up to your attic and then quiet your inner voices. Begin to inhibit by thinking, *I am* not *tensing in my body.* Then think, *I am* not *lifting my neck.* Sustain this thought as you wait for your helper to move your neck back. (You will be using your neck extensor muscles to do this movement but not your head extensors, which pull your head backward on your neck.)

Once you begin, move your neck back so that your forehead is no more than an inch off the floor. Stop moving. Hold your neck back *for no more than fifteen seconds* as you continue inhibiting. Put your head down on the floor and rest.

Be sure not to move your neck more than an inch. Be sure not to tense your jaw or tongue as you lift. Be sure not to work your head extensors—the muscles that move your head backward on your neck. If you pull your head back as you lift, you will be seeing out across the room (Illustration G-1-2). If you do it correctly, you will continue to see the floor.

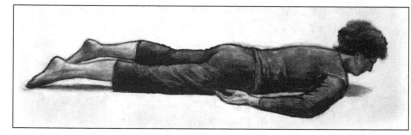

G-1-2. Prone: pulling the head backward on the neck, lifting the head off the floor by using the head extensors.

If you are not sure if you are using the right muscles, place a hand on the back of your neck and head as you did in section B-1. *As you lift, you should not feel your head moving backward on your neck, but you will feel muscles working to lift your neck.* You can also place the back of your hand on your lower back to gather information about what you are doing in this area. *You should not feel any tension in your lower back.*

3. Repeat the movement, using the skills you have gained thus far in these experiments: Quiet your voice and rise up to your attic. Take a moment to be clear about the movement, and then think of *not* moving. Wait for your helper. Continue thinking of *not* moving as you lift your neck back a little more. Stop. Sustain your inhibiting. If you are having success, then move your neck back one more inch. Stop. Sustain your thinking. Then put your head down on the floor and rest.

If at any point you feel muscles tensing that should not be tensing, put your head on the floor and rest, and then start again as you think of not lifting.

When you return your head to the floor, you may feel muscles letting go in other areas of your body. This means that you used these muscles as you lifted your neck, even though you did not feel them working when you did the movement. Now that you know this, the next time you try the movement, take more time to inhibit these muscles so that *you are only using the neck extensors.* Also, pay attention to your breathing. If you hold your breath, or tighten around your rib cage so that your ribs cannot move, you are tensing muscles that you should not use. Rest on the floor again and inhibit.

Try this movement just a few times, and then stop. Then pay attention to how your back feels the next day. If there is any ache in your neck or back muscles, especially in the lower back, wait until you feel better before trying the movement again. *Once you can do this small movement without difficulty and without experiencing any discomfort the following day, practice it each day, slowly increasing the number of repetitions and the length of time that you sustain the lift. You should not do more than about ten lifts, and do not hold each lift for more than about thirty seconds.*

▶ **DISCUSSION**

The *extensor muscles* of your torso are in your back. They extend from the back of your head to the bottom of your spine. As we have learned, most people do not use these muscles properly to support them upright, but instead let their spine collapse in a slouch; or they overwork the superficial muscles in the back, pulling themselves back and downward. Many people also tense too much in the muscles in the front of the neck and torso, which compounds the downward pulls on the spine. This situation is made even worse by muscle tension at the back of the head, which pulls the head's weight back and downward into the spine. The result of this is that the neck moves sharply forward from the upper chest, and the head is carried in front of the body. (See Illustrations II-1 and 1-1.) In this circumstance the *head extensors*—the muscles that pull the head back on the neck—are too tense. And the *neck extensors*—the muscles that support the neck so that it stays back, aligned with the rest of the spine rather than jutting forward—are weak.

In short, if your habit is to sit and stand with your neck jutting forward, your head pulled back, and your chest rounded forward, the deep *extensor muscles of the back* that run the full length of your spine are not working well. In the next exercise you will increase the neck lift by also moving your upper back off the floor. This is more difficult, so you need to do this slowly and with conscious inhibition and direction.

Before you try it, some words of caution. As we have discussed, while learning to use and strengthen these specific muscles, you should not use any unnecessary muscles. In particular, you should not tighten your head extensors and pull your head back. You should not tense the muscles of your buttocks or your hamstrings at the back of your thighs. You should not use muscles around your chest and ribs, or your shoulder or arm muscles. You should not hold your breath, tense your jaw, or strain anywhere in your body. In both exercises it is essential to move slowly and just a little bit at a time. Success is not measured by how far or how quickly you move.

Many people find these exercises difficult. If you have not used these muscles for a long time, when you try to do this you are likely to feel that it is impossible. Do not give up. Since you have not been using these muscles, your brain has not been activating the neural pathways that connect to them. Your brain will not immediately be able to figure out how to do the movement. Be patient, and practice for just a few minutes each day. Even if you do not move, taking time to ask your mind to *conceive* of the movement will help you progress in the right direction. Gradually, your helper will establish the right pathway, and one day you will find yourself able to do it.

Please read the instructions and the following discussion before beginning.

Neck and Back Extensors

[Note: If you have a neck injury, or neck or shoulder pain, do not try this without the assistance of an Alexander teacher.]

1. Lie in prone. Place your hands on the floor over your head with palms down, elbows bent, and upper arms away from your sides.

Quiet your voices, rise up to your attic and think, *I am not lifting my neck*. Then think the directions, *up, wide,* and *forward,* and *forward and up.*

Sustain your inhibiting and directing as you let your helper move your neck back with the neck extensor muscles. Stop moving and inhibit and direct. Move again. Stop. Inhibit and direct. Move a little farther. Continue in this way until you are lifting your head, neck, and upper spine, and your chest begins to lift off the floor (Illustration G-2-1).

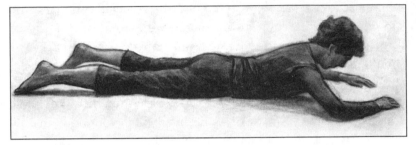

G-2-1. Prone: lifting the neck, head, and upper chest off the floor using the neck and back extensors and without pulling the head back, or tensing the muscles of the lower back.

You may find it more comfortable to do this movement without any books under your chest.

In this exercise you are simply continuing from the previous exercise. You are lifting your neck (and your head), and now your upper spine off the floor. Stop and inhibit frequently. Then move again about an inch. If you tense muscles that you do not need to use, stop and return to the floor. Rest. Restore your inhibiting and directing and try again. Be sure not to use shoulder or arm muscles, or press your hands into the floor.

If you are weak in your upper back muscles but tight in the muscles in the front of your neck and the front of your chest (*flexors*), this exercise will be difficult. Practice it for a short time each day, and only move as far as you can without tensing unnecessarily. Be patient. It may take several months, but gradually you will be able to lift your neck back, and lift your upper chest off the floor. (See Illustration 3-2: the first picture in the series on the left. This is one of the earliest movements that babies practice.)

2. Sit in a chair. Place your feet on the floor and your hands on your thighs. Think of quieting your voices and rise up to your attic. Think,

I am not sitting. Think, *I want my neck to move slightly back, my head to release forward and up, my back to lengthen up and widen, and my knees to release forward.*

Are you sitting differently than usual? Do you notice your back muscles working now to support your neck and head, and to connect your neck with your upper back? Are you lightly poised, balancing upright easily as you sit?

With inhibition, you are preventing your old habit of tension and collapse. With direction, you are engaging the deep muscles of your back to support your head, neck, and spine upright easily and efficiently.

H SELF-MASTERY EVERY DAY

> Our life is what our thoughts make it.
> —MARCUS AURELIUS ANTONINUS

This section offers instruction on how to use inhibiting and directing in your daily life. Specifically, it shows how these skills can help you exercise or play a sport more efficiently and skillfully, improve technical skills such as playing an instrument, enhance performance, and reduce harmful chronic conditions such as pain and anxiety. The conclusion of this section offers ideas for using inhibition and direction in a wide range of activities and circumstances, showing how these skills can enhance how you function in everything you do.

As you continue to practice, keep in mind that inhibiting and directing cannot always produce instantaneous or precisely predictable results that last for a specific period of time. You are learning to develop your powers of mind, journeying into an exploration of the nature of consciousness. This is a learning process, which means continuous change. As your skills increase, they will produce new results, which in turn will increase your skill, and so on. This process of growth will always include a little unpredictability, surprise, and a bit of mystery. After all you are not a machine. You cannot always perform the same.

In addition, keep in mind that this learning process has no completion. Your skills can always continue to deepen, yielding fresh insights and discoveries. Your objective is not to get to the end but to continue to apply what you are learning to all the acts of living. I hope that in addition to your growing self-understanding and self-mastery, you will enjoy a deepening sense of wonder at the power and potential within you.

Exercise

Do you exercise, either by working parts of your body (for example, lifting weights) or by doing a more whole body activity such as walking, jogging, biking, or swimming? These are excellent opportunities to apply your skills.

For example, if you want to lift a weight in your hand: Stop before you rush into your repetitions. Bring your attention to what you are doing and how you are thinking. No mind wandering. Rise up to your attic and think, *I am not lifting this weight.* Then think, *up, wide, and forward.* Add the thought *forward and up.* Renew the thought, *I am not lifting.* Wait for your helper. Continue thinking of not lifting as you renew your directions. Sustain this as you lift and also as you lower the weight.

You may discover that when you add inhibiting and directing, you cannot readily lift the same weight as before. This is a good sign. By inhibiting, you are preventing excess muscle tension. By directing, you are integrating your many-tiered locomotor system to coordinate the muscles of your entire body as you lift. This means you are *not* using muscles that are inappropriate for the task. Your new cognitive skills are also a barometer for letting you know when you are ready to lift more weight, and when you have done enough. Do not mindlessly lift the weight until you have reached a predetermined number of repetitions, or until your muscles give out. Lift the weight only as long as you can continue inhibiting and directing, integrating yourself as a whole as you move. You will be much less likely to injure yourself.

Do you jog? Before you begin, remind yourself that you want to think about how you are running. Do not go for a run while leaving your mind behind! Before you begin take a few minutes to inhibit with the thought, *I am* not *running.* You may feel muscles letting go that you did not know you used, or notice that muscles have already begun to tense in readiness for running. Think, *I do* not *want to tense my neck.* Direct, thinking, *I want to let my head release forward and up on my spine. I want to let my back lengthen upward and widen. I want to let my knees release forward.* Pay attention to sustaining your directing as you begin to run. Are you running differently? As you become more skilled with directing while you run, you will not have to say these instructions to yourself all the time. After a few repetitions, your mind will know what you want. If you notice at some point that your new psychophysical coordination has deteriorated, it means you are tiring. Stop running and walk for a short time. Once you can inhibit and direct easily again, resume running.

Do you bike? If you use drop handlebars, biking can be especially hard on your neck and back. The lowered hand position requires you to curve forward in your spine and then pull your head back, compressing your neck in order to see ahead of you. This means you are creating excessive tension in your flexor muscles and your head extensors—just the muscles you have been learning *not* to use. Unless you are racing competitively, I recommend that you change your handlebars so that they are level and your hand position is higher. This will allow your spine to maintain its length—from tail to head—as you pivot your body forward from your hip joints (as you practiced in section F-2). It also lets your arms extend away from your body as they lengthen toward the handles. Now you do not have to curve forward in your spine and pull your head back on your neck. Sitting more upright may feel wrong, but if you want to prevent neck injuries and keep riding your bike into old age, this is the way to do it.

As you ride, be aware of all the areas of contact between your body and the bike: handles, seat, and pedals. Think spatially to help you lengthen your body out and away—through your arms and hands out toward the handlebars, through your legs and feet out toward the pedals, through your spine to lengthen your back and send your pelvis into the seat. Riding a bike should be a bit like rock climbing. Beginning climbers usually tense too much, shortening their muscles and essentially pulling their hands and feet away from the rock face. Skilled climbers think of lengthening—toward their hands and toward their feet—lengthening their body outward into the rock. Although it feels less secure, it is more efficient and more effective.

Similarly, as a biker, you do not want to contract your muscles too much, making yourself hunch forward and down onto your bike, tensing your belly, and gripping the handlebars. This will subtly pull your body away from your bicycle. Instead, think of telling yourself *not* to clutch, and *not* to pull your head back. Then direct, thinking up, wide, and forward, and forward and up. Use your spatial thinking to create a quality of expansion throughout your whole body, especially as your leg muscles push against the resistance of the pedals. Think of your body expanding in space, outward in all directions toward your head, pelvis, feet, and hands.

Sports

If you play a sport that involves hitting, catching, or chasing a moving object, your most essential skill is seeing the object—and learning to recognize when you are not seeing it and then being able to recover it. Although most coaches can recognize when a player is not "keeping his eyes on the ball," they are usually unable to help a player learn to do this consciously and reliably. If you play this type of sport, I recommend that you reread chapter 13—the story of how I taught Jared to inhibit in order to see the ball.

To review, the essential point is that although you are in some sense seeing the object because your eyes are open, your mind is primarily focused elsewhere: You may be trying to feel your body and know what these feelings mean in order to make your muscles move your body in the right way. You may have your mind on trying to move your body faster/harder/farther/better. You may be worrying whether you are doing it right/going to win/making a mistake. You may be trying to remember your coach's instructions. You may also be trying too hard to see the object by overtensing muscles that control the movement of your eyes, and so fixing them on the object for a split second—by which time the object has moved on and you have lost it.

Invent your own variations on the experiment I did with Jared that are appropriate for your sport. Put down your bat, racket, stick, etc., and practice seeing the object moving toward you and past you. Notice if it mysteriously disappears from view. Although your eyes may be open, this means you are no longer seeing the object. Use your inhibition as you remind yourself not to try to see by tensing your eye muscles or your neck muscles. These must be loose to allow your eyes to move and your head to turn freely as the object you are watching travels through space. Do not try to see specific qualities of the object, or focus on its surface. Watch it moving. This requires that you also direct, so that you are seeing while sustaining an awareness of the space through which the object is traveling. As your ability to watch the object improves, increase the difficulty of the task by returning to the field and watching it as you deal with the other players, and think of the bigger aspects of the game.

Practice and Performance

If you have problems with performance anxiety, inhibition can be especially helpful. It can also help you improve your technique. Do you find yourself nervously anticipating an upcoming performance, anxious thoughts filling your mind as you worry that you will not perform well? Whenever you notice yourself thinking such worried thoughts, or just feeling generally anxious, it is time to inhibit. Think, *I am not performing*. Or, *I am not getting ready to perform*. If you spend sufficient time with this, you may experience an unfamiliar feeling of emptiness. This is the absence of your anxiety. It means that your inhibition is being successful. Unfortunately, performers often mistakenly believe this unfamiliar feeling means that they are not ready to perform. But it only means that you are not creating your anxiety. Although performers usually say that they do not like the feeling of performance anxiety, they often believe that anxiety is necessary to ensure a good performance. As a result, they subtly retrigger their anxiety. Ask yourself if this belief underlies your worry habit. Challenge your belief by taking time every day to think of not performing—even though the absence of your anxiety may feel strange—and discover for yourself that you can perform without it.

What happens when you practice difficult passages of music, prepare a long monologue, or practice a complicated dance combination? Notice how your attention narrows downward as you leave your attic to focus on the parts of your body. Notice your breathing. Notice your neck jutting a bit more forward, your shoulders and arms tensing. Notice your worry and effort. Stop. Think of *not* playing/acting/dancing. Bring your attention up to your attic, away from the page or your muscles. Think of space: up, wide, forward. Aim your thinking forward and up. Continue inhibiting and directing as you begin again. Make your inhibiting and directing your first priority. If you make a mistake, stop. Wait. Inhibit and direct. Begin again. If you find yourself feeling anxious because you have not yet made a mistake, stop. Think of *not* playing/acting/dancing. Direct and then begin again. In this way you can gradually free yourself from your habit of narrowing your mental focus, tensing your muscles too much, and feeding your worry habit. In time, you may find that that your overall coordination improves, that you have better balance and ease throughout your body, and that your problem has disappeared.

Anxiety

A student comes to me complaining that he has a problem with anxiety. "I have heartburn. I worry a lot. Every funny feeling in my body makes me think that this time there is something serious. It used to be a small problem. But each year it gets worse."

Comments such as these are not unusual. More and more people come to me in a state of chronic anxiety, and they are younger and younger. Sadly, my students seldom understand the bind they have created within themselves. Part of the problem stems again from erroneous beliefs, particularly about the meaning of bodily sensation. The more peculiar and uncomfortable the sensations, the more they believe that they are suffering from something serious. They know that these troubling feelings are happening more and more, and that they are worrying more and more. But they do not doubt the basic premise that is fueling the problem—their belief that something is wrong. Like Betty in chapter 5, most people never doubt their beliefs. They believe they are right to be worried. They believe that their worry is a rational and logical response to the conviction that there is something seriously wrong. In their mind, it is the feeling that happens first, and this causes the "rational" worry that follows from it. As long as they feel bad, how can they stop worrying?

In fact, it is not that there is a funny feeling, and as a result the student becomes worried. It is that the student is in a chronic condition of worry, which produces an array of odd physical sensations. As a result of this, his mind invents reasons to explain these feelings. And the more that his mind fills in the blank—it might be cancer or some other serious condition—the more this triggers his amygdala, which produces ever more neurochemical change that creates these strange feelings. As long as the student believes he is right to be worried, he will not conquer his worry habit.

Thus, at a low level of unconscious processing, our brain discerns the state of our organism (anxious). At a higher level of processing, our brain notices strange bodily experiences (feelings) and creates a story to explain them. (I must have a serious illness.) We would truly be trapped in this cycle if it were not for the fact that we have an even higher level of brain function. We can learn to understand what is happening within us: We can consciously appreciate how we are perpetuating our worry habit by believing in all of our mind's self-invented reasons for worrying. This highest level of brain activity comes to us through our prefrontal cortex. It is an override switch. With our prefrontal cortex, we can inhibit, thinking, *I do not have to be worried. I do not have to believe in my beliefs. This is only my mind's invention, a guess, a filling in of the blank. I can tell myself not to keep thinking this way. I can tell myself that every time a new, seemingly rational explanation comes into my mind I do not have to believe it. I do not have to perpetuate my mind-body anxiety with more fearful thinking.*

This takes practice and perseverance, and it requires taking time to think in this new way, but gradually inhibition can reverse the seemingly irreversible problem of a growing worry habit.

Pain

The challenge for people in chronic pain is similar to those in chronic anxiety, who often overfocus on their feelings. Recent research is showing that chronic pain seems to alter neural connections in the brain. As a result of chronic pain, the brain learns to become more pain sensitive and more pain perceptive. Feelings that other people might describe as "disturbing" or "uncomfortable," the chronic pain patient often describes as painful, sometimes severely so. In other words, more and more types of bodily sensations seem to be interpreted by the brain as meaning "pain."

This is usually accompanied by the individual's strongly held belief that the pain must be closely scrutinized, and that everything possible must be done to manage and avoid it. Like Ed in chapter 8, such people often lead diminished lives as they accumulate an ever longer list of activities that they believe cause their pain or make it worse. They become more and more fearful. If this psychophysical condition continues long enough, such people become a complex mixture of real pain, perceived pain, fear, and altered neurochemistry that compounds their chronic fear, fear behaviors, and faulty beliefs. Typically, they have been to many health specialists before they try an Alexander teacher, often as a last resort. Having experienced so much failure, and so many experts who have not been able to help them, they are skeptical of and unwilling to trust the teacher.

Inhibiting can be especially difficult for such students, because it seems completely wrong to them to be asked to lessen their attention on their pain. This flies in the face of their belief that they must focus on their pain in order to manage it. But if such students continue their lessons, when they progress to directing they may experience sudden improvement. Since chronic pain often creates a distortion in the mind's capacity to think spatially, by learning to think up, wide, and forward for brief periods throughout their day, they may experience a surprising reduction in their symptom.

How You Live

With your new skills you can create an infinite variety of self-experiments using inhibiting and directing as you engage in more complex physical and interpersonal activities. Here are some examples:

- **Inhibit and direct as you drive in traffic.** Think, *I am* not *driving; I am thinking up, wide, and forward.*
- **As you work at your desk think,** *I am* not *writing (or typing). I am* not *tensing my arms and legs. I am* not *holding my breath. I am* not *pulling my neck down. I am thinking up, wide, forward. I am directing forward and up.*
- **As you stand at the tee, ready to take your backswing before hitting the golf ball, stand in position for a few moments longer as you think,** *I am* not *swinging the club.* As you look at the ball, remind yourself to think of letting your neck be back, letting your head be forward and up, letting your knees release forward, and connecting your heels into the ground. Sustain your attention on directing and on seeing the ball, as you make the backswing and then through the entire downswing.

- **As you sit with your family at the Thanksgiving table, try thinking of quieting your inner voices.** Simply be present and quiet, and listen as others speak.

Try your new skills under circumstances in which you might not expect them to be helpful:

- **When your boss or spouse makes a thoughtless remark and you feel anger welling up within you,** tell yourself not to hold on to this emotion, and not to replay the incident again and again in your mind. Then think up, wide, and forward.
- **When your teenager tells you s/he hates you,** instead of yelling back (attacking—a fear response), tell yourself that you do not have to respond instantly. Stop. Think of *not* reacting. Think of your head releasing forward and up, your back lengthening up and widening, your knees releasing forward. Now consider what you want to say in response.
- **When a friend invites you to try something you have never tried before** (for example, an Alexander lesson), instead of quickly declining because of the low-level discomfort you feel as you imagine doing something that is unknown to you, remind yourself that your feelings are only momentary. How you feel now is not necessarily how you will feel later. Remind yourself that you do not know what this experience will be like, and you do not have to react instantly to these uneasy feelings by declining (withdrawal). Think, *I do not know what this will be. I do not have to assume I will not like it.* Then think, *up, wide,* and *forward* for a moment. Ask yourself again whether or not you want to try it. Maybe you will decide to change your mind.
- **When you are feeling mentally confused or tired,** instead of reaching for another cup of coffee, a drink, a cigarette, or a piece of chocolate, find a place to lie down in semisupine. Quiet your voices. Rise up to your attic—think up—and turn on your prefrontal cortex. Think with clarity of meaning: *I don't have to push on. I can take a moment and let my mind have a rest.* Continue inhibiting until you notice the thought rising in your mind, *I want to get up.* Then get up and carry on with what you were doing.

- When you are having a heated political argument with someone and are convinced of the rightness of your position, instead of repeating your argument again and again, becoming more and more frustrated and angry, make your point and then stop speaking. Wait. Allow yourself to become aware of yourself. Notice the position you are sitting in. Notice the room around you. Notice the person you are speaking to. Notice your breathing. Notice the feeling of tension in your neck. Think, *I am* not *tensing*. Think, *I do* not *have to win this argument*. Think, *I am expressing my opinion, but I might not be entirely right*. Think, *I want to quiet my voices, and suspend my beliefs, so that I can better listen to the other person's point of view and try to understand it.*
- Inhibit when you have not been able to do something successfully. Stop and wait. Then try again.
- Lie in semisupine or prone and take time to inhibit when you experience emotions that are overwhelming to you.
- When you are engaged in a creative project that requires imaginative and innovative thinking but ideas are not coming to you, instead of pushing yourself harder and harder, becoming more and more determined to get it done, lie down in semisupine frequently. Inhibit and rest your mind. Wait. Trust that as you rest, your helper will do the thinking for you. You may be surprised to find that new insights and ideas arise in your mind spontaneously.

How to Find a Teacher

FOUNDED IN 1987, the American Society for the Alexander Technique (AmSAT) maintains the profession's highest standards for teacher training, certification, professional conduct, and membership. The Society is affiliated with fourteen national societies around the world that share these standards.

AmSAT-certified teachers have been trained in an AmSAT approved, three-year teacher training course that consists of 1,600 class hours over a minimum of three years, with a five-to-one student-teacher ratio. Alternatively, individuals not trained in an AmSAT course may receive certification through application to AmSAT for individual review and evaluation.

To find an AmSAT-certified teacher, please visit AmSAT's website at: www.AmSAT.ws, or call (800) 473-0620.

AmSAT's website provides a national membership directory, a list of teacher training courses nationwide, contact information for the affiliated societies, and a calendar of upcoming events and workshops. It also offers for sale a comprehensive line of books, CDs, DVDs, and other items on the Technique. AmSAT invites the public to join the Society as Associate Members who receive such benefits as AmSAT's quarterly newsletter. You can visit the AmSAT office at 30 North Maple Street, Florence, MA 01062.

For a directory of non-AmSAT teachers, contact Alexander Technique International at: www.ati-net.com.

ANXIETY The wide-ranging effects (mental and physical, conscious, and unconscious) on an individual produced by chronic activation of the amygdala.

APPRAISAL The amygdala's evaluation of sensory stimuli for threat to the organism.

ASSOCIATIVE TRIGGER A harmless stimulus that occurs in connection with a threatening stimulus, which the amygdala learns to associate with danger and so, over time, also interprets as threatening.

ATTENTION A capacity of the mind to focus on a particular thought, stimulus, feeling, or action while lessening its focus on other thoughts, stimuli, feelings, or actions. The mind can shift attention consciously or unconsciously. Attention is a mental skill that can be consciously practiced and improved.

ATTIC This is a metaphor for the prefrontal cortex. The term "rise up to the attic" refers to the ability to consciously learn to better activate the prefrontal cortex to enhance conscious inhibitory skill.

AWARENESS A capacity of the mind that enables us to perceive ourselves, and then to perceive more and more sensory stimuli, both from within and outside the self, simultaneously. Awareness is a mental skill that can be consciously practiced and improved.

BELIEF A judgment the mind forms from bodily sensations. (I am not using this word to refer to religious ideas or convictions.) As such, beliefs are the mind's interpretation of sensory experience. Beliefs are usually unconscious but may become conscious. They may also be inaccurate or incorrect. Beliefs may be changed and become more accurate through improving our locomotor skill, which changes sensory feedback.

BIPEDALISM The human locomotor strategy, which involves carrying the head on top of a vertically aligned spinal column that is poised on top of two straightened hind limbs. In walking or running, the non–weight-bearing forelimbs (arms) swing in counterbalance to the alternately weight-bearing and striding hind limbs (legs).

BODILY SENSATION I refer to this as our sixth sense, defined as the wide spectrum of sensory inputs that inform the brain about the state, condition, and actions of the psychophysical organism. This sensory system includes inputs that are proprioceptive (from muscles and joints) and interoceptive (from the viscera). Bodily sensations can be received and processed by the brain entirely below the level of conscious awareness, or they can be semiconscious, or they can be made increasingly conscious. The brain may misinterpret the meaning of bodily sensations. It can also learn to more accurately interpret their meaning. I use this term synonymously with *feeling*. I include awareness of our emotional states as coming to us via this sensory system.

BRACHIATOR A vertebrate locomotor strategy that involves using the arms to support the body by holding on to overhead supports (branches), and traveling through space by hanging and swinging from one support to another.

DIRECTING I define directing as spatial thinking, a mental capacity we derive from our vestibular apparatus that enables us to perceive three-dimensional space and to conceive of specific directions in space. Directing is a mental capacity that we can consciously learn to enhance. Directing plays a role in improving balance and toning the deep muscles of the spine to coordinate the torso in a headward direction.

END-GAINING Focusing one's attention exclusively on a particular result or outcome without regard for or with insufficient attention to the best means of achieving it.

EXPANDING FIELD OF AWARENESS This term refers to the teacher's skill, as s/he is touching the student, of becoming increasingly aware of sensory inputs from both his/her body and the student's body simultaneously.

FAULTY SENSORY APPRECIATION This is Alexander's term for the mind's tendency to misjudge or misinterpret bodily sensation.

FIGHT-OR-FLIGHT RESPONSE The organism's innate mechanisms for perceiving threat and behaving in self-defense. This term can be misleading, however, since it implies that our defense response is either to run away or to fight. In fact, animals have four stereotyped defense behaviors: attack, withdraw, freeze, and submit.

HABITUAL WAY OF MOVING A learned and unconscious pattern of muscle activity that enables us to perform specific acts. Once we learn to hold a pen and write, for example, we think, *write,* and our brain coordinates our muscles in a characteristic pattern. We are not usually conscious of how we have learned to do this, and so we cannot easily change our habitual way of moving.

HELPER This metaphor refers to subcortical areas of the brain (especially the cerebellum) that play a key role in helping to smoothly coordinate our muscles in activity, enabling us to move with greater efficiency and skill.

INHIBITION, INHIBITING At a neurological level, inhibition is the capacity of a neuron to cause another neuron to be less easily activated. In the Alexander Technique, conscious inhibition is a skilled use of the mind to prevent or cease unwanted, harmful, or unnecessary behavior as it is happening or as it begins.

INITIATING TRIGGER A stimulus that the amygdala appraises as threatening, causing it to trigger the organism into defense behavior.

INTENTION A formulation in the mind of a desired aim.

LOCOMOTOR SYSTEM The system of muscles, bones, joints, nerves, etc., that enables an animal to move parts of itself and also to move its entire body from place to place.

MISUSE A harmful, inefficient, or ineffective way of moving or using the self (mind and body), which is generally unconscious.

MOTOR NERVES Nerves that stimulate a muscle to contract.

NEUROCHEMICAL RESPONSE The neurological and chemical changes that are caused once the amygdala appraises a stimulus as threatening.

NON-DOING Another term for inhibition.

PREFRONTAL CORTEX The most frontal area of the cerebral cortex, and the most recently evolved area of the brain. Scientists are learning that this region performs an executive function, integrating and overseeing the behavior of the whole individual, and especially for exerting inhibitory or impulse control.

PRIMARY CONTROL Alexander defined this as a dynamic relationship between the head and neck, and between the head, neck, and trunk that enhances the individual's locomotor coordination and its overall functioning.

PROPRIOCEPTION Charles Sherrington coined this term (perception of one's own) to refer to the sensory capacity that is derived from sensory receptors in our muscles, tendons, and joints, including the vestibular apparatus, which inform the brain of the body's movements in space. I have proposed that proprioception be considered a subset of a broader sixth sense of bodily sensation, and that this sixth sense exclude the vestibular apparatus, which would be better classified as a discrete sensory system.

QUADRUPED A vertebrate locomotor strategy that involves carrying the trunk horizontally on top of four limbs, the feet leveraging against the ground to propel the animal in the direction of its head.

REACTION An unnecessary, harmful, inappropriate, maladaptive, or inefficient response to a stimulus. Reactions may be described as primarily physical or mental, but they involve the whole organism.

SELF A construct of the mind, made possible by the cortex and especially the prefrontal cortex, that assimilates information from all the sensory systems, but especially from bodily sensations, and creates a construct that we speak of as "I."

SELF-DEFENSE SYSTEM All the structures of the organism that enable it to evaluate a sensory stimulus for danger, and then to propel the organism into behaviors of defense.

SEMIBRACHIATOR A vertebrate locomotor strategy that involves supporting the body largely with the two hind limbs, with the torso positioned diagonally or semi-upright on the hind limbs, and the arms and knuckles of the hands used for partial weight bearing.

SENSORY FEEDBACK I use this synonymously with bodily sensation, but it can be used more broadly to refer to sensory inputs from any of our sensory systems.

SENSORY RECEPTORS A broad term that refers to the many types of specialized sense organs and nerve endings located throughout the body that are sensitive to a particular type of stimulus and cause sensory nerves to fire.

SENSORY STIMULI Inputs received by the brain from sensory nerves.

SOMATOSENSORY CORTEX An area of the cerebral cortex in the brain that processes sensory inputs from the body, giving us the capacity to become consciously aware of bodily sensations or feelings.

STEREOTYPED DEFENSE BEHAVIORS Vertebrates have four unlearned and stereotyped behaviors in response to real or perceived danger: freeze, attack, withdraw, and submit. These behaviors range from overt behaviors to neurochemical changes that cannot be felt or perceived.

SYMPATHETIC NERVOUS SYSTEM Together with the parasympathetic nervous system, these comprise the *autonomic nervous system,* which largely controls the activity of the internal organs. Broadly speaking, the sympathetic system arouses the organism, preparing it for activities involving strength, energy, and action. The sympathetic nervous system is aroused by the amygdala to activate the organism into behaviors of defense.

VESTIBULAR APPARATUS A sensory structure located on both sides of the head and close to the inner ear, consisting of three semicircular, fluid–filled canals and the utricle and saccule. This sensory system enables us to think spatially and directionally, informs us of the direction of gravity and the direction of movement of the head, and plays a part in helping us to balance upright, coordinate muscle tone (especially of the trunk), and to orient our movements in space.

INTRODUCTION TO THE ALEXANDER TECHNIQUE

1. Magnus. "Some Results of Studies in the Physiology of Posture, Part I." 1926, p. 536.
2. Among Alexander's students at the time were Sir Henry Irving and Viola Tree.

CHAPTER THREE

1. Dart. "Voluntary Musculature of the Human Body: The Double-Spiral Arrangement." 1950, pp. 265–68.
2. For more on our adaptations to bipedalism: Tobias. *Man, The Tottering Biped.* 1982.

CHAPTER FOUR

1. There are fascinating accounts of infants who were lost in forests in Europe in the 1800s, reared by wolves, and who then later recovered. Intriguingly, these children didn't learn to stand upright and walk as bipeds, but clambered about on all fours. For more on this: Lane. *The Wild Boy of Aveyron.* 1976.

CHAPTER FIVE

1. For more on recent neurological research into the link between reasoning and bodily experience: Damasio. *Descartes' Error: Emotion, Reason and the Human Brain.* 1994.

CHAPTER SEVEN

1. For more on this: LeDoux. *The Emotional Brain.* 1998.
2. Ibid, p. 131.

CHAPTER EIGHT

1. For more on the effects of stress hormones on neurological functioning: LeDoux. *The Emotional Brain*. 1998.
2. Schwartz and Begley. *The Mind and The Brain: Neuroplasticity and the Power of Mental Force.* 2002, p. 218.

CHAPTER TWELVE

1. Alexander. *The Use of the Self.* 1932, pp. 3–36.
2. Binkley. *The Expanding Self.* 1993, p. 95.
3. Ibid, p.104.
4. Ibid, p. 93
5. Goldberg. *The Executive Brain: Frontal Lobes and the Civilized Mind.* p. 35–36: "The prefrontal cortex is directly interconnected with every distinct functional unit of the brain. It is connected to the posterior association cortex, the highest station of perceptual integration. . . . In addition, this command

post connects with the amygdala. . . . Of all the structures in the brain, only the prefrontal cortex is embedded in such a richly networked pattern of neural pathways. This unique connectivity makes the frontal lobes singularly suited for coordinating and integrating the work of all the other brain structures—the conductor of the orchestra. . . . Indeed, experiments have shown that the concept of 'self,' which is deemed to be a critical attribute of the conscious mind, appears only in the great apes. And it is only in the great apes that the prefrontal cortex acquires a major place in the brain."

6. Schwartz and Begley. *The Mind and The Brain: Neuroplasticity and the Power of Mental Force.* 2002. p. 312: "Without inflating the philosophical implications of this and similar findings, it seems safe to conclude that the prefrontal cortex plays a central role in the seemingly free selection of behaviors, choosing from a number of possible actions by inhibiting all but one and focusing attention on the chosen one. It makes sense, then, that when this region is damaged patients become unable to stifle inappropriate responses to their environment: a slew of possible responses bubbles up, as it does in all of us, but brain damage robs patients of the cerebral equipment required to choose the appropriate one."

7. Kotulak. *Inside The Brain: Revolutionary Discoveries of How The Mind Works.* 1996, p. 69.

8. Society for Neuroscience. Brains and Briefings: "Serotonin and Judgment," 2002, http://apu.sfn.org.

9. The Associated Press, "Scientists Discover Musicians' Brains Are Wired Differently." 2001.

10. Begley. "Parts of the Brain that Get Most Use Literally Expand and Rewire on Demand," 2001, p. B1.

11. Leuchter. "Changes in Brain Function of Depressed Subjects During Treatment with Placebo." 2002. Also: Vedantam. "Against Depression, A Sugar Pill is Hard to Beat." 2002.

CHAPTER FIFTEEN

1. Shainberg. "Finding the Zone." 1989.

CHAPTER EIGHTEEN

1. To give one recent example of this common oversight, in *Scientific American*'s latest Special Edition, December 2006, the cover is titled, "Secrets of the Senses: How the brain deciphers the world around us." Beneath this title is a list of our senses: "vision, smell, hearing, touch, and taste."

2. In addition, your brain learns about the *rate of speed* of the movement of your head by the rate of firing of these hairlike cells.

3. Berthoz. *The Brain's Sense of Movement.* 2000, p. 132

4. LeDoux. *The Synapse.* 2003, p. 303: "The neural mechanism underlying the perception of spatial relations is present in both hemispheres of other primates; it is mainly on the right side in humans. This implies that spatial perception was forced from the left during the language invasion of human synaptic territory."

CHAPTER TWENTY

1. Wolkomir. "Charting the Terrain of Touch." 2000.

2. Wilson. *The Hand.* 1999.

3. Napier. *Hands.* 1993, p. 55.

Achenbach, Joel. "You Feel That?" *National Geographic*, January 2005

Alexander, F. M. *Articles and Lectures.* London: Mouritz Press, 1995.

_____. *Man's Supreme Inheritance,* 6th ed., New York: E. P. Dutton and Co., 1941.

_____. *Constructive Conscious Control of the Individual.* London: Methuen and Co., 1924.

_____. *The Universal Constant in Living.* New York: E. P. Dutton, 1941.

_____. *The Use of the Self.* New York: E. P. Dutton, 1932.

Begley, Sharon. "How Mirror Neurons Help Us To Empathize, Really Feel Others' Pain." *The Wall Street Journal*, March 4, 2005.

_____. "Maybe for This Year, You Can Try Whipping Your Brain Into Shape." *The Wall Street Journal,* October 29, 2002.

_____. "Parts of the Brain That Get Most Use Literally Expand and Rewire On Demand." *The Wall Street Journal,* October 11, 2001.

Bernstein, N., Mark Latash, ed., Michael Turvey, ed. *Dexterity and its Development.* Mahwah, NJ: Lawrence Erlbaum Assoc., 1996.

Berthoz, Alain. *The Brain's Sense of Movement.* Cambridge: Harvard University Press, 2000.

Binkley, Goddard. *The Expanding Self: How The Alexander Technique Changed My Life.* London: STAT Books, 1993.

Bloch, Michael. *F.M.: The Life of Frederick Matthias Alexander.* London: Little, Brown, and Co., 2004.

Bramble, Dennis, and Daniel Lieberman. "Endurance Running and the Evolution of Homo." *Nature*, November 18, 2004.

Candia, Victor, and Christian Wienbruch, Thomas Elbert, Brigitte Rockstroh, William Ray. "Effective Behavioral Treatment of Focal Hand Dystonia In Musicians Alters Somatosensory Cortical Organization." *Proceedings of the National Academy of Science* 100, no. 13 (2003).

Chase, Marilyn. "Yogi Berra Was Right." *The Wall Street Journal,* October 29, 2002.

Damasio, Antonio. *Descartes' Error.* New York: G. P. Putnam's Sons, 1994.

_____. *The Feeling of What Happens.* New York: Harcourt, Brace and Jovanovich, 1999.

Dart, Raymond. "Voluntary Musculature in the Human Body: The Double-Spiral Arrangement." *The British Journal of Physical Medicine* 13, no. 12 (1950).

Garlick, D., ed. *Proprioception, Posture, and Emotion.* New South Wales: CPME, 1982.

Goleman, Daniel. "Early Violence Leaves Its Mark On The Brain." *New York Times,* October 3, 1995.

Groopman, Jerome. "Hurting All Over." *The New Yorker,* November 13, 2001.

_____. "When Pain Remains." *The New Yorker,* October 10, 2005.

Hobson, J. Allan. *The Chemistry of Conscious States.* Boston: Little, Brown, and Co., 1994.

Kalb, Claudia. "Coping With Anxiety." *Newsweek,* February 24, 2003.

Kotulak, Ronald. *Inside the Brain: Revolutionary Discoveries of How The Mind Works.* Kansas City: Andrews and McMeel, 1996.

Kuriyama, Shigehisa. *The Expressiveness of the Body and the Divergence of Greek and Chinese Medicine.* New York: Zone Books, 1999.

Lane, Harlan. *The Wild Boy of Aveyron.* Cambridge: Harvard University Press, 1976.

LeDoux, Joseph. *The Emotional Brain.* New York: Simon & Schuster, 1996.

_____. *Synaptic Self: How Our Brains Become Who We Are.* New York: Penguin Group, 2003.

Lemonick, Michael. "Glimpses of Consciousness." *Time,* July 17, 1995.

Leonard, Jonathan. "The Sorcerer's Apprentice." *Harvard Magazine,* May–June 1999.

Leuchter, A., and I. A. Cook, E. A. Witte, M. Morgan, and M. Abrams. "Changes in Brain Function of Depressed Subjects During Treatment With Placebo," *American Journal of Psychiatry* 159, no. 1 (2002).

Libet, Benjamin. "Neural Destiny." *The Sciences* 29, no. 2 (1989).

Magnus, Rudolph. "Some Results of Studies in the Physiology of Posture, Part I." *The Lancet,* September 11, 1926.

Malin, Shimon. *The Eye That Sees Itself.* Sandpoint, ID: Morning Light Press, 2004.

Mann, J. John. Brain Briefings "Serotonin and Judgment." *Society for Neuroscience,* April 1997, http://apu/sfn.org. .

Mead, Nathaniel. "Mind/Body Answer to Allergies." *Natural Health,* September 1995.

Napier, John. "The Evolution of the Hand," *Scientific American* 707, no. 6 (1962).

Nathan, Peter. *The Nervous System.* Oxford: Oxford University Press, 1988.

Ornstein, Richard, and Richard Thompson. *The Amazing Brain.* Boston: Houghton Mifflin Co., 1984.

"Pain Perception: Mind Tricks." *The Economist,* August 27, 2005.

Reid, Brian. "The Nocebo Effect: Placebo's Evil Twin." *Washington Post,* April 30, 2002.

Rogers, Adam. "The Brain: Thinking Differently." *Newsweek,* December 7, 1998.

Sacks, Oliver. "A Neurologist's Notebook: Speed." *The New Yorker,* August 23, 2004.

Schommer, Nancy. *Stopping Scoliosis: The Complete Guide to Diagnosis and Treatment.* Garden City Park, NY: Avery Publishing Group, 1991.

Schwartz, Jeffrey M., and Sharon Begley. *The Mind and The Brain: Neuroplasticity and The Power of Mental Force.* New York: Regan Books, 2000.

"Scientists Discover Musicians' Brains Are Wired Differently." *Daily Hampshire Gazette,* November 15, 2001.

Shainberg, Lawrence. "Finding The Zone," *New York Times Magazine,* April 9, 1989.

Sherrington, C. S. *The Integrative Action of the Nervous System.* New Haven: Yale University Press, 1906.

Smetacek, Victor. "Mind-grasping Gravity." *Nature* 415 (2002).

Smetacek, Victor and Franz Mechsner. "Making Sense." *Nature* 432 (2004).

Sternberg, Esther, and Philip Gold. "The Mind-Body Interaction in Disease." *Scientific American,* Special Edition, 2002.

Thernstrom, Melanie. "My Pain, My Brain." *New York Times Magazine,* May 14, 2006.

Tobias, Philip. *Man, the Tottering Biped: The Evolution of his Posture, Poise and Skill.* Kensington, NSW, Aust.: CPME, 1981.

Vedantam, Shankar. "Against Depression, A Sugar Pill Is Hard To Beat." *Washington Post,* May 7, 2002.

Wade, Nicholas. "Improved Scanning Technique Uses Brain As Portal To Thought." *New York Times,* April 25, 2005.

Wilson, Frank R. *The Hand.* New York: Vintage Books, 1999.

Wolkomir, Richard. "Charting the Terrain of Touch," *Smithsonian,* June 2000.

FURTHER READING ON THE ALEXANDER TECHNIQUE

Balk, Malcolm, and A. Shields. *The Art of Running.* London: Ashgrove, 2000.

Cacciatore, Tim, Fay Horak, and Sharon Henry. "Improvement in Automatic Postural Coordination Following Alexander Technique Lessons in a Person With Low Back Pain." *Physical Therapy* 85) no. 6 (2005).

Carrington, Walter. *Thinking Aloud: Talks on Teaching the Alexander Technique.* Edited by Jerry Sontag. San Francisco: Mornum Time Press, 1994.

Cranz, Galen. *The Chair.* New York: W. W. Norton, 1998.

Dart, Raymond. *Skill and Poise.* London: STAT Books, 1996.

De Alcantara, Pedro. *Indirect Procedures: A Musician's Guide to the Alexander Technique.* Oxford: Clarendon Press, 1997.

Dewey, John. "Introduction," *Constructive Conscious Control of the Individual,* 8th ed., by F. M. Alexander, London: Chaterson, Ltd., 1946.

_____. "Introduction," *The Use of the Self,* by F. M. Alexander, New York: E. P. Dutton, 1932.

_____. "Introductory Word," *Man's Supreme Inheritance,* 6th ed., by F. M. Alexander, New York: E. P. Dutton, 1941.

Heirich, Jane. *Voice and the Alexander Technique: Active Explorations for Speaking and Singing.* San Francisco: Mornum Time Press, 2005.

Huxley, Aldous. *Ends and Means.* New York: Harper and Brothers, 1937.

Jones, Frank P., Florence Gray, John Hanson, and D. N. O'Connell. "An Experimental Study of the Effect of Head Balance on Patterns of Posture and Movement in Man." *Journal of Psychology* 47 (1959).

Jones, Frank P. *Body Awareness in Action.* New York: Schocken Books, 1976.

_____. "Method for Changing Stereotyped Response Patterns by the Inhibition of Certain Postural Sets," *Psychological Review* 72 (1965).

Langford, Elizabeth. *Mind and Muscle: An Owner's Handbook.* Apeldorn, Netherlands: Garant Uitgevers, 1998.

Machover, Ilana, and A. and J. Drake. *The Alexander Technique Birth Book: A Guide to Better Pregnancy, Natural Birth and Parenthood.* London: Robinson, 1993.

Shaw, Steven, and Armand D'Angour. *The Art of Swimming: In a New Direction with the Alexander Technique.* Bath, UK: Ashgrove Publishing, 1996.

Stallibrass, Chloe, P. Sissons and C. Chalmers. "Randomized Controlled Trial of the Alexander Technique for Idiopathic Parkinson's Disease." *Clinical Rehabilitation* 16 (2002).

Tinbergen, N. "Ethology and Stress Diseases." *Science I* 185 (1974).

FROM THE GERM of an idea to a book in hand, this has been a ten-year project. Such a task has not been the work of myself alone. The list of people to whom I owe a debt of gratitude is long. I can repay them only in small measure with this mention.

My thanks and deep appreciation to friends, colleagues, students, and others who read the manuscript in part or in whole, during one phase of the project or throughout, and shared their thoughts, suggestions, and encouragement: Cynthia Knapp, Charlotte Lemann, Peggy and Murray Schwartz, Tully Hall, Carol Vineyard, Steph Bouffard, Jeannie Guillet, Judy Stern, Idelle Packer, Christine Stevens, Christine Olson, Jerry Sontag, Jean Fischer, Tova and Shimon Malin, Priscilla Hunt, Katarina Hallonblad, Jimmy Helling, Margaret Boyko, Ruth Rootberg, Jeff Korff, Shellie Steuer, Wendy Woodson, Michael Bloch, Eric Kay, Joe Levinski, Chloe Stallibrass, Mary Flesher, James Shreeve, Phyllis Richmond, Sara Belchetz-Swenson, Robin Maltz, Jennifer Gates, Cherida Lally, Polly Ehrgood, Julia Ehrgood, Emily Ehrgood, Kitty Benedict, Peter Anderheggen, Michaela Hauser-Wagner, Paul Recker, and Heather Strizalkowski.

For modeling for the illustrations, which frequently meant holding their body in tight positions for long periods, my deep appreciation to: Priscilla Hunt, Margaret Boyko, Katarina Hallonblad, Sara Miller, and Tom Ehrgood.

Publishing a book by a first-time author, on a complex subject that many people have never heard of before, requires special people to take it from first draft to public eye. Beverly Martin at AR&E gave me the first validation that publishing was not a pipe dream. Ellie Lipman reached out to her many contacts on my behalf and opened my eyes to the world of agents, publishers, publicists, and contracts. Mark London read a stranger's book proposal and not only expressed his wholehearted enthusiasm but also recommended it to his agent. My gratitude and thanks go to Rafe Sagalyn and his hardworking assistant Eben Gilfenbaum for believing in (and being patient with) an untested author, and recognizing that the word needed to get out. I have been incredibly fortunate to find a home for my labors with the kind-spirited, patient, and skillful Matthew Lore at Marlowe & Company, and his hardworking and committed team. They have translated ideas into form and beauty.

Lucy Brown, elegant neuroscientist, gave up her limited free time to read a manuscript by someone she had never met and give invaluable feedback, as well as her approbation to a nonscientist's effort to bring neuroscience to Alexander's discoveries.

I was enormously lucky to find and then work with Matt Mitchell, the book's extraordinary illustrator. It was an exciting time in the project when, as I joined Matt in his studio, his charcoal and eraser in hand, we discussed the nuances of light, shade, and form to puzzle out how to highlight the subtle qualities of use and misuse in the drawings. His superb illustrations stand above all others in showing the mind-body in action among books on the Alexander Technique.

Many have said that family members of authors ought to receive more public recognition. This author's family is no exception. My brother, John Vineyard, gave his sister needed encouragement at a crucial juncture, persuading me—joined by the vociferous enthusiasm of friend Peter Bouffard—that the book should be adapted for a wider audience. My wonderful sons, Jared and Jules, endured with patience many late dinners and a distracted mother, and provided source material for the book. The spirit of my parents, Phyllis and George Vineyard, shone through late at night when I thought I must be nuts, and told me not to quit.

Finally, I owe an inestimable debt to my husband, Tom, who arrived unexpectedly at my doorstep one evening to take me to dinner at just the moment I had concluded that dating and book writing were completely incompatible, swept me off my feet, and proposed five weeks later. Our wedding slowed the writing process, but I would not have a published book without him nor would it be as well written.

INDEX

A

acting, stage, 277–284,
  299–300
Alexander Technique
  development of, 7–12
  overview, 2
Alexander, Frederick
  Matthias, 7
amygdala, 73–76, 81, 85
anatomy, evolution of, 27–34
anxiety, 76, 300–301
  mind/body connection,
    81–82, 95, 122, 140
  performance anxiety,
    91–94, 96, 99–103,
    299–300
athletes, 178–179, 298–299
  baseball, 128–136,
    190–191
  helper and, 148
attention, 102, 115–119
attention deficit disorder
  (ADD), 113–114, 115
attic, mental, 115–121
  finding, 155–157
  thinking from, 157–159
awareness, 94, 192, 247–250,
  257

B

back
  injuries, 42
  muscles, 31, 41–48
  pain, 23–26, 37, 137–144,
    207, 270–276

strengthening, 289–295
balance, 193–196, 202–209,
  217. *see also* vestibular
  apparatus
baseball, 128–136, 190–191
basement, mental, 119
beliefs, 59–63, 96–97, 140, 286
  anxiety and, 300–301
  conscious inhibition and,
    171
  letting go, 69–70,
    172–174
  pain and, 268
  placebo effect, 125
biking, 297–298
Binkley, Goddard, 112
bipedalism, 26, 29, 37
bodily sensation/feedback,
  57–63, 286
  belief and, 69–70
  defense behavior and,
    75–76, 88–90
  inability to notice, 66–67
  misjudgments, 145, 215
  problems with, 165,
    191–196
  touch, 238
body lightness, 107–110,
  270–276
brachiators, 28
brain
  amygdala, 73–74, 81, 85
  frontal lobes, 113
  operating systems of,
    146–147

prefrontal cortex, 113,
115–116, 118, 125,
155–159

C

Carrington, Walter, 107
center of gravity, 31, 32
conscious choice, 97–98
conscious inhibition, 103–104,
110, 118, 126, 151
avoiding no, 162–166
experiments, 166–174
feeling/thinking, 154–159
meaning and, 159–162,
167
quiet inner conversation,
152–153, 167
controlling impulses, 113
coordination, 206–209, 217

D

daily living skills, 295–304
Damasio, Hanna, 114
dancing, 299–300
danger, 73–76
defense behaviors, 74
bodily sensation and,
75–76, 81–82, 88–90,
140
changing, 97–98
pain and, 266, 268
psycholocomotor system
and, 86
stress hormones, 84–85
defensive messaging, 87–88
depression, 124–125, 235–237
directing
Alexander's directions,
225–227
conscious, 211, 216
defined, 4, 10, 202

experiments for, 217–227
in daily life, 295–304
moving with, 228–232
teaching process and,
213–215, 249, 253–260
disconnection, 252

E

emotions, 58, 70, 95
evolution, 27–34, 146–147
exercise, 24, 145, 296–298
expanding field of awareness,
247–250, 257

F

facial muscles, 87–88
facial pain, 210–212
fear, 71–76, 77–80, 95, 103, 140,
268–269
feeling(s), 95, 154–159,
191–196, 238. *see also* bodily
sensation/feedback
fibromyalgia, 83–85, 96
field of awareness, 94, 247–250,
257
fight-or-flight response, 74
freeze behavior, 140

H

habits of mind, 151
avoiding no, 162–166
chasing mental butterflies,
152–154
feeling instead of thinking,
154–159
loss of meaning, 159–162
habits of misuse, 114
habitual way of moving, 3
head position, 11
helper, 133, 136, 142, 147
experiments for, 170–172

hip pain, 67–70, 212–215
hyperactivity disorder (HD),
   113–114

I

impulses, controlling, 113
inhibition, 121
   attic and, 118
   back pain, 144
   defined, 3, 10
   in daily life, 295–304
   moving with, 228–232
   teaching process and, 115,
      138–142, 146, 249,
      253–260
injury, 266
intention, 119
interoception, 58

J

jogging, 296–297

K

knowing-by-feeling, 121, 192

L

language, 181, 208, 286
locomotor functioning, 206
locomotor systems, 24
   bipedalism, 26, 29, 33, 37
   evolution of, 27–34
   muscles of, 30–31
   pain and, 266
   primary, 36
   quadruped, 28, 36

M

Mangus, Rudolf, 11
meaning, 239
   loss of, 159–162

self reflection and, 94
   summoning, 161–162
   thinking with, 160, 167
mental butterflies, chasing,
   152–154
mental skills
   positive no, 164–167
   quiet inner conversation,
      152–153, 167
   think with meaning,
      160–162, 167
   turn on prefrontal cortex,
      155–159, 167
mind/body connection, 9–11,
   95–96, 102, 215
   anxiety, 93, 101, 122
   bodily sensation, 57–63
   disconnection, 12
   misjudgments, 70, 145
   pain and, 268
   placebo effect, 125
   self-observation, 53–54
misuse, habits of, 9, 114, 252–253
motion, 48–54, 198
motor nerves, 74
moving
   with inhibition and
      direction, 168–169,
      228–232
muscle(s), 10, 31, 206
   back, 30, 31, 32, 41–48,
      289–295
   strength, 24, 145
musculoskeletal injuries, 42
musculoskeletal system
   see locomotor system

N

neck, 42, 43–44, 290–295
nervous system, 74

neurochemical responses, 74
neurons, 10
numbness, leg, 23–26

O

orienting-by-directing, 192
osteoporosis, 77

P

pain, 301–302
    back, 23–26, 37, 137–144,
        207, 270–276
    chronic, 85
    defense behavior and, 266,
        268
    facial, 210–212
    hip, 67–70, 212–215
    shoulder, 17–22, 37, 207,
        263–269
panic attacks, 78
performance anxiety, 91–94, 96,
    99–103, 299–300
practice and performance,
    299–300
prefrontal cortex, 113, 125
    attic and, 115–116, 118
    finding the attic, 155–157
    thinking from the attic,
        157–159, 167
principle of non-doing, 112. *see
    also* inhibition
prone position, 42, 45–48
proprioception, 58, 198, 205
psycholocomotor system, 35,
    86
psychophysical function, 70,
    144, 146, 224, 252, 287

Q

quadruped(s), 28, 36–37

R

reflexes, 11
rest positions, 41–48
rigidity, 269
Ritalin, 114
running, 39

S

self awareness, 19, 48–54, 58, 94,
    149, 286–288
self-experiments, 13–14
    conscious inhibition,
        168–174
    directing, 217–227
    mind and motion, 48–54,
        228–232
    spatial thinking, 218–224
semibrachiators, 28
semicircular canals. *see* vestibular
    apparatus
semisupine position, 42–45
sense of feeling. *see* bodily
    sensation
sensory feedback, 61, 126
    conscious inhibition and,
        171
    errors in, 70, 86, 189
sensory receptors, 57, 154, 238
shoulder
    injuries, 42
    pain, 17–22, 37, 207,
        263–269
sleeping positions, 42
somatosensory cortex, 85, 147
spatial thinking, 182–188, 208,
    211
    awareness, 192, 206
    experiments for, 218–224
    orienting, 201–202
    pain and, 268

speaking techniques, 279–284
spinal stenosis, 23–26
spine, 31
sports, 298–299
    baseball, 128–136, 190–191
stress, 84–85, 123, 126
students
    Betty, hip pain, 67–70,
        212–215
    Brian, facial pain, 210–212
    Bruce, performance
        anxiety, 91–94, 99–103
    Ed, fibromyalgia, 83–85
    Erin, back pain, 23–26, 37,
        137–144, 207, 270–276
    Gary, lack of awareness,
        64–67
    Greg, acting, tension,
        277–284
    Jim, fear, 80
    Joan, fear, 77–80
    John, shoulder pain, 17–22,
        37, 207, 263–269
    Meghan, introverted teen,
        187–188, 208
    Nancy, balance, 193–196,
        204

Nathan, baseball, 190–191
Sam, depression, 235–237
supra sensory system, 286
sympathetic nervous system, 74

T
teaching process
    expanding field of
        awareness, 247–250, 257
    getting plugged in, 246
    summary, 259–260
tension, 208, 269, 277–284
touch, 237–244, 251–260
triggers, fear, 103

V
vertebrae, neck, 43
vertigo, 200–202, 203
vestibular apparatus, 33, 197,
    198–202. *see also* balance

W
weightlifting, 39, 296